KETO DIET COOKBOOK

for Women over 50

ULTIMATE GUIDE FOR SENIORS, GET RID OF LOWER BELLY FAT FEMALE, LOSE WEIGHT, BALANCE HORMONES, EASY KETOGENIC DIET RECIPES, DAYS MEAL PLAN

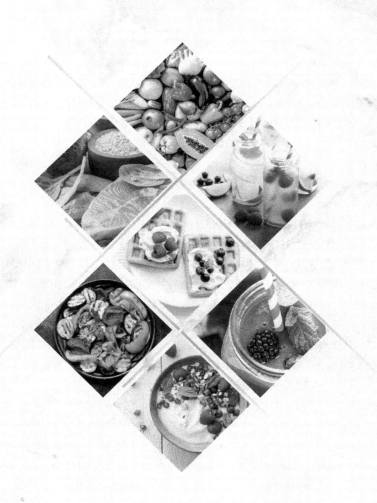

Winifred Campbell

TABLE OF CONTENTS

Introduction   11

1. Baked Cream Cheese Muffins   14

2. Bacon and Egg Avocado Breakfast Wrap   15

3. Kale Salad with the Bacon and Blue Cheese   16

4. Greek Salad with Vinaigrette Salad Dressing   17

5. Bacon Avocado Salad   18

6. Cauliflower, Shrimp, and Cucumber Salad   19

7. Seared Squid Salad with Red Chili Dressing   20

8. Cauliflower and Cashew Nut Salad   21

9. Salmon and Lettuce Salad   22

10. Prawns Salad with mixed Lettuce Greens   23

11. Poached Egg Salad with Lettuce and Olives   24

12. Beef Salad with Vegetables   25

13. Niçoise Salad   26

14. Shrimp, Tomato, and Avocado Salad   27

15. Cauliflower Mash   28

16. Buttery Garlic Steak   29

17. Baked Lemon Salmon   30

18. One Sheet Fajitas   31

19. Balsamic Chicken   32

20. Pesto Chicken Salad   33

21. Fresh Summer Salad   34

22. KETO TACO SALAD   35

23. MIXED VEGETABLE TUNA SALAD   36

24. SAUSAGE AND CHEESE PUFFS   37

25. FROZEN BERRY BITES   38

26. CREAM CHEESE AND HAM ROLLS   39

27. KETO-FRIENDLY CRACKERS   40

28. KETO ICE CREAM   41

29. CHEESECAKE FAT BOMBS   42

30. LEMON BARS   43

31. KETO BAKED SALMON WITH LEMON AND BUTTER   44

32. KETOGENIC SPICY OYSTER   45

33. GARLIC LIME MAHI-MAHI   46

34. FISH AND LEEK SAUTÉ   47

35. SMOKED SALMON SALAD   48

36. KETO BAKED SALMON WITH PESTO   49

37. ROASTED SALMON WITH PARMESAN DILL CRUST   50

38. KETO FRIED SALMON WITH BROCCOLI AND CHEESE   51

39. KETO RIB EYE STEAK   52

40. BACON BLEU ZOODLE SALAD   53

41. GARLIC BAKED BUTTER CHICKEN   54

42. LEMON ROSEMARY CHICKEN THIGHS   55

43. COFFEE BUTTER RUBBED TRI-TIP STEAK   56

44. KETO GROUND BEEF AND GREEN BEANS   57

45. SPICY BEEF MEATBALLS   58

46. CHILLED CUCUMBER SOUP   59

47. CREAMY MUSHROOM SOUP   60

48. BROCCOLI SOUP   61

49. MEATBALLS SOUP   62

50. SHRIMP WITH ASPARAGUS   63

51. SHRIMP CURRY   64

52. SEAFOOD STEW   65

53. TOMATO & MOZZARELLA SALAD   66

54. CUCUMBER & TOMATO SALAD   67

55. CHICKEN & BROCCOLI CASSEROLE   68

56. TURKEY CHILI   69

57. BEEF CURRY   70

58. SHEPHERD'S PIE   71

59. PORK WITH VEGGIES   72

60. PORK TACO BAKE   73

61. SHRIMP LETTUCE WRAPS   74

62. CHICKEN STUFFED AVOCADO   75

63. CHICKEN & VEGGIE SKEWERS   76

64. STUFFED TOMATOES   77

65. CRAB CAKES   78

66. PEPPERONI PIZZA   79

67. BACON WITH MUSHROOMS   80

68. SHRIMP WITH ZUCCHINI NOODLES   81

69. SPINACH WITH COTTAGE CHEESE   82

70. GREEN CHICKEN CURRY   83

71. CREAMY PORK STEW   84

72. SALMON & SHRIMP STEW   85

73. CREAMY CHICKEN BAKE   86

74. BEEF & VEGGIE CASSEROLE 87

75. BEEF WITH BELL PEPPERS 88

76. COCONUT KETO PORRIDGE 89

77. CREAM CHEESE EGGS 90

78. CREAMY BASIL BAKED SAUSAGE 91

79. KETO BRUNCH SPREAD 92

80. MUSHROOM OMELET 93

81. 1-MINUTE KETO MUFFINS 94

82. PEANUT BUTTER PROTEIN BARS 95

83. TUNA STUFFED AVOCADO 96

84. BACON BURGER CABBAGE STIR FRY 97

85. BACON CHEESEBURGER 98

86. CAULIFLOWER MAC & CHEESE 99

87. MUSHROOM & CAULIFLOWER RISOTTO 100

88. SKILLET CABBAGE TACOS 101

89. CHICKEN-PECAN SALAD & CUCUMBER BITES 102

90. CURRY EGG SALAD 103

91. KETO-CAULI TOTS 104

92. SPICY SAUSAGE AND PORTOBELLO PIZZA'S PLANS 105

93. CHICKEN AND PROSCIUTTO SALAD WITH ARUGULA AND ASIAGO 106

94. CAESAR BRUSSELS GROWS WITH ALMONDS SALAD. 107

95. CHICKEN PAN-GRILLED WITH CHORIZO CONFETTI 108

96. SALMON WITH PESTO, RED PEPPER 109

97. LEMONY SHRIMP GRILLED PLATE OF MIXED GREENS 110

98. ROASTED RED PEPPER AND CHICKEN 111

99. SAUSAGE PATTIES WITH SPINACH 112

100. BROILED SALMON AND ASPARAGUS WITH CRÈME FRAICHE 113

101. Flank Steak Skillet Barbecued	114
102. Avocados stuffed with Crap	116
103. Blackened Chicken Salad	117
104. Vinaigrette with Blue Cheese	118
105. Mint Raita grilled Chicken with Tandoori	119
106. Salmon Salad with Feta Cheese	120
107. Spicy Shrimp Salad	121
108. Keto Mustard Salad	122
109. Warm Kale Salad	123
110. Broccoli Salad with Dill	124
111. Collagen Mug Cake	125
112. Chocolate and Nut Butter Cups	126
113. Peanut Butter Cup Chaffle	127
114. Cinnamon Sugar Chaffle	128
115. Cinnamon and Cream Cheese Chaffle	129
116. Golden Chaffles	130
117. Churro Chaffle	131
118. Yogurt Chaffle	132
119. Zucchini Chaffle	133
120. Cauliflower Chaffle	134
121. Zesty Chili Lime Tuna Salad	135
122. Sheet Pan Brussels Sprouts and Bacon	136
123. Super Simple Chicken Cauliflower Fried Rice	137
124. Prep-Ahead Low-Carb Casserole	138
125. BBQ Pulled Beef Sando	139
126. Keto-friendly Oatmeal Recipe	140
127. Crunchy Coconut Cluster Keto Cereal	141

128. Avocado Egg Bowls   142

129. Keto Cinnamon Coffee   143

130. Keto Waffles and Blueberries   144

131. Baked Avocado Eggs   145

132. Mushroom Omelet   146

133. Chocolate Sea Salt Smoothie   147

134. Zucchini Lasagna   148

135. Vegan Keto Scramble   149

136. Parmesan Cheese Strips   150

137. Peanut Butter Power Granola   151

138. Homemade Graham Crackers   152

139. Keto no-Bake Cookies   153

140. Swiss Cheese Crunchy Nachos   154

141. Keto Cheesecake with Blueberries   155

142. Keto Lemon Ice Cream   156

143. Peanut Butter Balls   157

144. Classic Pork Tenderloin   158

145. Signature Italian Pork Dish   159

146. Flavor packed Pork Loin   160

147. Spiced Pork Tenderloin   161

148. Sticky Pork Ribs   162

149. Valentine's Day Dinner   163

150. Southeast Asian Steak Platter   164

151. Pesto flavored Steak   165

152. Flawless grilled Steak   166

153. Mongolian Beef   167

154. SICILIAN STEAK PINWHEEL   168

155. AMERICAN BEEF WELLINGTON   169

156. PASTRY-FREE BEEF WELLINGTON   170

157 SUPER SALMON PARCEL   171

158. NEW ENGLAND SALMON PIE   172

159. KETO SAUSAGE BREAKFAST SANDWICH   173

160. CABBAGE HASH BROWNS   174

161. KETO BREAKFAST CUPS   175

162. EGG SALAD RECIPE   176

163. BUFFALO SHRIMP LETTUCE WRAPS   177

164. BROCCOLI BACON SALAD   178

165. KETO BACON SUSHI   179

166. CAPRESE ZOODLES   180

167. ZUCCHINI SUSHI   181

168. BASIL AVOCADO FRAIL SALAD WRAPS & SWEET POTATO CHIPS   182

169. CALIFORNIA BURGER BOWLS   183

170. PARMESAN BRUSSELS SPROUTS SALAD   184

171. KETO QUESADILLAS   185

172. KETO STUFFED CABBAGE   186

173. GARLIC ROSEMARY PORK CHOPS   187

174. LEMON BUTTER FISH   188

175. CHILI LIME COD   189

176. LEMON GARLIC SHRIMP PASTA   190

177. ONE-PAN TEX MEX   191

178. SPINACH ARTICHOKE-STUFFED CHICKEN BREASTS   192

179. Chicken Parmesan — 193

180. Sheet Pan Jalapeño Burgers — 194

181. Grilled Herb Garlic Chicken — 195

182. Blackened Salmon with Avocado Salsa — 196

183. Delectable Tomato Slices — 197

184. Grain-free Tortilla Chips — 198

185. Cheeses Chips — 199

186. Snack Parties Treat — 200

187. Sweet Tooth Carving Pana Cotta — 201

188. Halloween special Fat Bombs — 202

189. Breakfast Toast in a Bowl — 203

190. Cocoa and Berry Breakfast Bowl — 204

191. Turmeric Nut Loaf with Zesty Cream Cheese — 205

192. Herby Goat Cheese Frittata — 206

193. Chocolate American Pancakes — 207

194. Green Shakshuka — 208

195. Eggs and Cheddar Breakfast Burritos — 209

196. Cheesy Guacamole with Veggie Sticks — 210

197. Cheese Patties with Raspberry Dip — 211

198. Tempura Zucchinis with Cream Cheese Dip — 212

199. Cheese Fondue with Low-Carb Croutons — 213

200. Cold Avocado & Green Beans Soup — 214

Conclusion — 215

Introduction

When you start at about 50, you will notice a lot of changes in your body, it is more than normal. Among the most common symptoms there is loss of muscle, insomnia, finer skin. You don't have to worry about this. Still, you have to pay much more attention than usual to your lifestyle, it is essential to keep fit, that you start attending a gym, as well as a healthy and correct diet under all macros.

You can apply it even if you even more effectively. But this is "something more," the information in this book is more than enough, you just have health problems. Of course, a visit to a nutritionist can help you personalize your diet need to study it and apply it diligently.

As said, the functions of our body change according to age, in particular, the thing that changes most is our metabolism, it is physiological that it slows down with age. This change is due both to aging but also to our lifestyle. Current metabolism is a consequence of our lifestyle in recent years.

A healthy lifestyle, with frequent, low-abundance meals, with moderate alcohol consumption, will certainly have a faster metabolism than a lifestyle consisting of large meals eaten once a day, alcohol, insomnia.

The ketogenic diet can help you from this point of view, eliminating carbohydrates and promoting the elimination of fats from our body. Another advantage is its flexibility, in fact, you can play with macros and adapt them to your needs and the way you live, in addition to the progress made, of course.

Start gradually, your body has adapted for years to an unhealthy lifestyle, so do not overdo it overnight. Take your time and slowly reach your goals. There is no need to run, this is a marathon, not 100 meters.

At first, you may feel tired, tired, without energy. Don't worry it's a normal thing, it's your body that is adapting to the new food style. You're taking away its basic source of energy, carbohydrates, it's logical that it has to adapt. It must change the main energy source, it must switch to using fats, but this takes time, two or three days are necessary. The drop in sugars could decrease your pressure for a couple of days, avoid exercise and there will be no problems. The resulting benefits will be enormous.

Here are some tips to get started:

1. Consult a nutrition specialist. This book is a very valuable tool to get an idea of what a ketogenic diet is, what the benefits are, how to avoid classic mistakes. It is a complete guide, with which, if studied well, you will certainly be able to set your diet according to your daily needs. However, consulting a doctor is never a bad idea, you can discuss your opinions and can give you valuable advice. I recommend consulting your doctor especially in cases of health problems and in cases where you have never been on a diet.
2. Take "fats" from unrefined foods (such as olive oil, avocado, walnuts). It has already been well said but I will never tire of repeating it: the quality of food is fundamental; you cannot think of obtaining concrete results (from any diet) if you do not eat quality food. Diets are based on scientific concepts, which give incredible results if you carefully follow the principles on which it is founded. It is not the magic wand, you will not lose weight from day to day, you will have to be persevering, even if not above all, in choosing the quality of the food.
3. Don't forget to eat starchy vegetables.
4. Don't overdo it with protein. Remember that we are always talking about a diet, so you will still have a certain calorie deficit. This will always true, but it is especially true for the ketogenic diet. Taking the right dose of protein is fine, taking a little more is not a problem, but taking a lot more yes. For two basis, the first and most important is that the body has a certain ability to assimilate proteins, if this is greatly exceeded, some organs, including the liver, may not function well. The second reason, if you do not create an energy deficit, you will never lose weight.
5. Drink and consume electrolytes (water, herbal teas, fresh juices). "taking on a little more isn't a problem?" Perfect, to be even more precise: taking a little more is not a problem IF taking the right amount of liquids. You can't do it differently, we should always drink a lot, but this is even more true in cases where we decide to follow a ketogenic diet: liquids are used by the organs to dispose of all proteins, if we don't drink, if we don't dilute proteins, the organs will suffer and we will have many other problems.

These are the 5 basic tips that you absolutely must follow, with constancy and diligence. For those who want to investigate further aspects in detail, from a scientific point of view.

1. Baked Cream Cheese Muffins

PREPARATION TIME: 10'	**SERVINGS:** 6
COOKING TIME: 12'	

INGREDIENTS

- 4 tablespoons melted butter, plus more for greasing the muffin tin
- ¾ tablespoon baking powder
- 1 cup almond flour
- 2 large eggs, lightly beaten
- 2 ounces (57 g) cream cheese mixed with 2 tablespoons heavy whipping cream
- A handful of shredded Mexican blend cheese

DIRECTIONS

1. Preheat the oven to 400°F (205°C). Grease 6 muffin tin cups with melted butter and set aside.
2. Combine the baking powder and almond flour in a bowl. Stir well and set aside.
3. Stir together 4 tablespoons melted butter, eggs, shredded cheese, and cream cheese in a separate bowl.
4. Add the dry mixture into the egg mixture, then using a hand mixer to beat until it is creamy and well blended.
5. Spoon the mixture into the greased muffin cups evenly. Bake in the preheated oven for about 12 minutes, or until the tops spring back lightly when gently pressed with your fingertip.
6. Remove from the oven and allow to cool for about 6 minutes, then serve warm.

NUTRITION: Calories: 298 Cal Fat: 20 g Carbs: 4 g Protein: 8 g Fiber: 3 g

2. Bacon and Egg Avocado Breakfast Wrap

| Preparation Time: | 10' | | Servings: | 2 |

| Cooking Time: | 10' |

Ingredients

- 6 bacon slices
- 2 large eggs
- 2 tablespoons heavy whipping cream
- 1 cup fresh spinach, chopped
- ½ avocado, sliced
- Pink Himalayan salt, to taste
- Freshly ground black pepper, to taste

Directions

1. Add the bacon slices to a large skillet over medium-high heat, and fry for 6 to 8 minutes until crispy, flipping occasionally.
2. With a slotted spoon, transfer the bacon to a paper towel-lined platter. Reserve the bacon grease in the skillet for later use.
3. Beat the eggs and heavy cream in a bowl, then add the salt and pepper. Stir well.
4. Slowly pour the egg mixture into the skillet with the reserved bacon grease, swirling the pan to spread evenly.
5. Cook for 1 minute, lifting the edges with a spatula to let the uncooked egg mixture flow underneath. Flip it over and cook for 1 minute more until set.
6. Fold one edge of the omelet over and slice in half, then transfer to two serving plates lined with paper towels, allowing the extra grease to soak up.
7. Make the wraps: Scatter each top with the cooked bacon, spinach, and avocado slices. Season with salt and pepper, then roll the wraps and serve.

Nutrition: Calories: 298 Cal Fat: 22 g Carbs: 5 g Protein: 3 g Fiber: 3 g

3. Kale Salad with the Bacon and Blue Cheese

Preparation Time: 10'

Servings: 2

Cooking Time: 10'

Ingredients

- 4 bacon slices
- 1 tablespoon vinaigrette salad dressing
- 2 cups fresh kale, stemmed and chopped
- Pinch pink Himalayan salt
- Pinch freshly ground black pepper
- ¼ cup pecans
- ¼ cup crumbled blue cheese

Directions

1. Add the bacon slices to a skillet over medium-high heat, and fry for 3 t0 4 minutes on each side until evenly crisp.
2. With a slotted spoon, transfer the bacon to a plate lined with paper towels. Set aside to cool.
3. In a large bowl, pour the vinaigrette over the kale and massage it into the kale with your hands. Season with salt and pepper, then allow standing for 5 minutes.
4. Make the salad: Chop the cooked bacon and pecans on your cutting board. Transfer them to the bowl of kale, and top with a sprinkle of blue cheese. Toss the mixture until well blended.
5. To serve, divide the salad between two serving plates.

Nutrition: Calories: 328 Cal Fat: 19.7 g Carbs: 5 g Protein: 8 g Fiber: 4 g

4. Greek Salad with Vinaigrette Salad Dressing

PREPARATION TIME:	10'		SERVINGS:	2

COOKING TIME:	0'

INGREDIENTS

- ½ cup halved grape tomatoes
- 2 cups chopped romaine lettuce
- ¼ cup feta cheese crumbles
- ¼ cup sliced black olives
- 2 tablespoons vinaigrette salad dressing
- Pink Himalayan salt, to taste
- Freshly ground black pepper, to taste
- 1 tablespoon olive oil

DIRECTIONS

1. Make the salad: Stir together the tomatoes, romaine lettuce, feta cheese, olives, and vinaigrette in a large bowl.
2. Sprinkle with salt and pepper, then pour over the olive oil. Toss the salad until well combined.
3. To serve, divide the salad between two serving bowls.

NUTRITION: Calories: 278 Cal Fat: 19.2 g Carbs: 4.6 g Protein: 7.3 g Fiber: 3 g

5. Bacon Avocado Salad

| Preparation Time: | 20' | Servings: | 4 |

| Cooking Time: | 0' |

Ingredients

- 2 hard-boiled eggs, chopped
- 2 cups spinach
- 2 large avocados, 1 chopped and 1 sliced
- 2 small lettuce heads, chopped
- 1 spring onion, sliced
- 4 cooked bacon slices, crumbled

Directions

1. In a large bowl, mix the eggs, spinach, avocados, lettuce, and onion. Set aside.
2. Make the vinaigrette: In a separate bowl, add the olive oil, mustard, and apple cider vinegar. Mix well.
3. Pour the vinaigrette into the large bowl and toss well.
4. Serve topped with bacon slices and sliced avocado

Nutrition: Calories: 268 Cal Fat: 16.9 g Carbs: 8 g Protein: 5 g Fiber: 3 g

6. Cauliflower, Shrimp, and Cucumber Salad

Preparation Time: 10'		**Servings:** 6
	Cooking Time: 15'	

Ingredients

- ¼ cup olive oil
- 1 pound (454 g) medium shrimp
- 1 cauliflower head, florets only
- 2 cucumbers, peeled and chopped

Directions

1. In a skillet over medium heat, heat the olive oil until sizzling hot. Add the shrimp and cook for 8 minutes, stirring occasionally, or until the flesh is pink and opaque.
2. Meanwhile, in a microwave-safe bowl, add the cauliflower florets and microwave for about 5 minutes until tender.
3. Remove the shrimp from the heat to a large bowl. Add the cauliflower and cucumber to the shrimp in the bowl. Set aside.
4. Make the dressing: Mix the olive oil, lemon juice, lemon zest, dill, salt, and pepper in a third bowl. Pour the dressing into the bowl of shrimp mixture. Toss well until the shrimp and vegetables are coated thoroughly.
5. Serve immediately or refrigerate for 1 hour before serving.

Nutrition: Calories: 308 Cal Fat: 19 g Carbs: 4 g Protein: 5 g Fiber: 3 g

7. Seared Squid Salad with Red Chili Dressing

Preparation Time: 10'

Servings: 4

Cooking Time: 5'

Ingredients

- 4 medium squid tubes, cut into rings
- 1 tablespoon chopped cilantro, for garnish

Salad:

- 1 cup arugula
- 2 medium cucumbers, halved and cut in strips
- ½ red onion, finely sliced
- ½ cup mint leaves
- ½ cup cilantro leaves, reserve the stems
- Salt and black pepper, to taste
- 2 tablespoons olive oil, divided

Directions

1. Make the salad: Mix the arugula, cucumber strips, red onion, mint leaves, and coriander leaves in a salad bowl. Add the salt, pepper, and 1 tablespoon olive oil. Toss to combine well and set aside.
2. Make the dressing: Lightly pound the red chili, garlic clove, and Swerve in a clay mortar with a wooden pestle until it forms a coarse paste. Mix in the lime juice and fish sauce. Set aside.
3. Warm the remaining olive oil in a skillet over high heat. Add the squid and sear for about 5 minutes until lightly browned.
4. Transfer the squid to the salad bowl and top with the dressing. Stir well. Serve garnished with the cilantro.

Nutrition: Calories: 278 Cal Fat: 24 g Carbs: 6 g Protein: 7 g Fiber: 5 g

8. Cauliflower and Cashew Nut Salad

Preparation Time: 10'

Servings: 4

Cooking Time: 5'

Ingredients

- 1 head cauliflower, cut into florets
- ½ cup black olives, pitted and chopped
- 1 cup roasted bell peppers, chopped
- 1 red onion, sliced
- ½ cup cashew nuts
- Chopped celery leaves, for garnish

Directions

1. Add the cauliflower into a pot of boiling salted water. Allow to boil for 4 to 5 minutes until fork-tender but still crisp.
2. Remove from the heat and drain on paper towels, then transfer the cauliflower to a bowl.
3. Add the olives, bell pepper, and red onion. Stir well.
4. Make the dressing: In a separate bowl, mix the olive oil, mustard, vinegar, salt, and pepper. Pour the dressing over the veggies and toss to combine.
5. Serve topped with cashew nuts and celery leaves.

Nutrition: Calories: 298 Cal Fat: 20 g Carbs: 4 g Protein: 8 g Fiber: 3 g

9. SALMON AND LETTUCE SALAD

PREPARATION TIME: 10'

SERVINGS: 4

COOKING TIME: 0'

INGREDIENTS

- 1 tablespoon extra-virgin olive oil
- 2 slices smoked salmon, chopped
- 3 tablespoons mayonnaise
- 1 tablespoon lime juice
- Sea salt, to taste
- 1 cup romaine lettuce, shredded
- 1 teaspoon onion flakes
- ½ avocado, sliced

DIRECTIONS

1. In a bowl, stir together the olive oil, salmon, mayo, lime juice, and salt. Stir well until the salmon is coated fully.
2. Divide evenly the romaine lettuce and onion flakes among four serving plates. Spread the salmon mixture over the lettuce, then serve topped with avocado slices.

NUTRITION: Calories: 271 Cal Fat: 18 g Carbs: 4 g Protein: 6 g Fiber: 3 g

10. Prawns Salad with mixed Lettuce Greens

Preparation Time: 10'

Servings: 4

Cooking Time: 3'

Ingredients

- ½ pound (227 g) prawns, peeled and deveined
- Salt and chili pepper, to taste
- 1 tablespoon olive oil
- 2 cups mixed lettuce greens

Directions

1. In a bowl, add the prawns, salt, and chili pepper. Toss well.
2. Warm the olive oil over medium heat. Add the seasoned prawns and fry for about 6 to 8 minutes, stirring occasionally, or until the prawns are opaque.
3. Remove from the heat and set the prawns aside on a platter.
4. Make the dressing: In a small bowl, mix the mustard, aioli, and lemon juice until creamy and smooth.
5. Make the salad: In a separate bowl, add the mixed lettuce greens. Pour the dressing over the greens and toss to combine.
6. Divide the salad among four serving plates and serve it alongside the prawns.

Nutrition: Calories: 228 Cal Fat: 17 g Carbs: 3 g Protein: 5 g Fiber: 8 g

11. Poached Egg Salad with Lettuce and Olives

PREPARATION TIME: 10'

SERVINGS: 4

COOKING TIME: 10'

Ingredients

- 4 eggs
- 1 head romaine lettuce, torn into pieces
- ¼ stalk celery, minced
- ¼ cup mayonnaise
- ½ tablespoon mustard
- ½ teaspoon low-carb sriracha sauce
- ¼ teaspoon fresh lime juice
- Salt and black pepper, to taste
- ¼ cup chopped scallions, for garnish
- 10 sliced black olives, for garnish

Directions

1. Put the eggs into a pot of salted water over medium heat, then bring to a boil for about 8 minutes.
2. Using a slotted spoon, remove the eggs one at a time from the hot water. Let them cool under running cold water in the sink. When cooled, peel the eggs and slice into bite-sized pieces, then transfer to a large bowl.
3. Make the salad: Add the romaine lettuce, stalk celery, mayo, mustard, sriracha sauce, lime juice, salt, and pepper to the bowl of egg pieces. Toss to combine well.
4. Evenly divide the salad among four serving plates. Serve garnished with scallions and sliced black olives.

NUTRITION: Calories: 261 Cal Fat: 17 g Carbs: 8 g Protein: 5.2 g Fiber: 3.16 g

12. Beef Salad with Vegetables

Preparation Time: 10'

Servings: 4

Cooking Time: 10'

Ingredients

- 1-pound (454 g) ground beef
- ¼ cup pork rinds, crushed
- 1 egg, whisked
- 1 onion, grated
- 1 tablespoon fresh parsley, chopped
- ½ teaspoon dried oregano
- 1 garlic clove, minced
- Salt and black pepper, to taste
- 2 tablespoons olive oil, divided

Salad:
- 1 cup chopped arugula
- 1 cucumber, sliced
- 1 cup cherry tomatoes, halved
- 1½ tablespoons lemon juice
- Salt and pepper, to taste

Directions

1. Stir together the beef, pork rinds, whisked egg, onion, parsley, oregano, garlic, salt, and pepper in a large bowl until completely mixed.
2. Make the meatballs: On a lightly floured surface, using a cookie scoop to scoop out equal-sized amounts of the beef mixture and form into meatballs with your palm.
3. Heat 1 tablespoon olive oil in a large skillet over medium heat, fry the meatballs for about 4 minutes on each side until cooked through.
4. Remove from the heat and set aside on a plate to cool.
5. In a salad bowl, mix the arugula, cucumber, cherry tomatoes, 1 tablespoon olive oil, and lemon juice. Season with salt and pepper.
6. Make the dressing: In a third bowl, whisk the almond milk, yogurt, and mint until well blended. Pour the mixture over the salad. Serve topped with the meatballs.

Nutrition: Calories: 302 Cal Fat: 13 g Carbs: 6 g Protein: 7 g Fiber: 4 g

13. Niçoise Salad

Preparation Time: 5'

Servings: 6

Cooking Time: 30'

Ingredients

- ¾ cup MCT oil
- ½ cup lemon juice
- 1 teaspoon Dijon mustard
- 1 tablespoon fresh thyme leaves, minced
- 1 medium shallot, minced
- 2 teaspoons fresh oregano leaves, minced
- 2 tablespoons fresh basil leaves, minced
- Celtic sea salt and freshly ground black pepper, to taste

Directions

1. Melt the butter and heat the olive oil in a nonstick skillet over medium-high heat. Place the tuna steaks in the skillet, and sear for 3 minutes or until opaque, flipping once. Set aside.
2. Make the dressing: Combine all the ingredients for the dressing in a bowl.
3. Make six niçoise salads: Dunk the lettuce and tuna steaks in the dressing bowl to coat well, then arrange the tuna in the middle of the lettuce. Set aside.
4. Blanch the green beans in a pot of boiling salted water for 3 to 5 minutes or until soft but still crisp. Drain and dry with paper towels.
5. Dunk the green beans in the dressing bowl to coat well. Arrange them around the tuna steaks on the lettuce.
6. Top the tuna and green beans with hard-boiled eggs, anchovies, avocado chunks, tomatoes, and olives. Sprinkle 2 tablespoons dressing over each egg, then serve.

Nutrition: Calories: 197 Cal Fat: 16 g Carbs: 8 g Protein: 6 g Fiber: 4 g

14. Shrimp, Tomato, and Avocado Salad

Preparation Time:	5'	**Servings:**	4

Cooking Time: 30'

Ingredients

- 1 pound (454 g) shrimp, shelled and deveined
- 2 tomatoes, cubed
- 2 avocados, peeled and cubed
- A handful of fresh cilantro, chopped
- 4 green onions, minced
- Juice of 1 lime or lemon
- 1 tablespoon macadamia nut or avocado oil
- Celtic sea salt and fresh ground black pepper, to taste

Directions

1. Combine the shrimp, tomatoes, avocados, cilantro, and onions in a large bowl.
2. Squeeze the lemon juice over the vegetables in the large bowl, then drizzle with avocado oil and sprinkle the salt and black pepper to season. Toss to combine well.
3. You can cover the salad, and refrigerate to chill for 45 minutes or serve immediately.

Nutrition: Calories: 158 Cal Fat: 10 g Carbs: 4 g Protein: 9 g Fiber: 3 g

15. Cauliflower Mash

Preparation Time: 10'

Servings: 4

Cooking Time: 5'

Ingredients

- 1 head cauliflower, chopped roughly
- ¼ cup heavy whipping cream
- ½ cup shredded Cheddar cheese
- 2 tablespoons butter, at room temperature
- Sea salt and freshly ground black pepper, to taste

Directions

1. Fill large saucepan three-quarters full with water and bring the water to a boil over high heat
2. Blanch the cauliflower in the boiling water for about 4 to 5 minutes, until it starts to soften.
3. Remove from the heat and drain on a paper towel.
4. Put the cauliflower to a food processor, along with the heavy cream, cheese, and butter. Process until it's creamy and fluffy. Sprinkle with the salt and pepper.
5. Divide the cauliflower mixture among four serving bowls, and serve

Nutrition: Calories: 148 Cal Fat: 16 g Carbs: 5 g Protein: 7 g Fiber: 4 g

16. Buttery Garlic Steak

| Preparation Time: | 10' | | Servings: | 4 |

| Cooking Time: | 30' |

Ingredients

- 1 lb. of steak
- 5 tbsp. of grass-fed butter
- 5 tbsp. of garlic cloves
- .25 cup of parsley
- A dash salt

Directions

1. One of the secret tips I can give you for the Ketogenic Diet is to put butter on absolutely everything that you can. Vegetable? Butter. Side dish? Butter. Main dish? Butter! This garlic butter steak is out of this world and incredibly easy to make. Before you even think about cooking, you will want to set aside several moments to season your steak properly. The best technique to use would be patting the steak down and then season with pepper and salt on both sides. Be generous with your seasoning!
2. Next, it is time to cook your steak. If you have a heavy-duty skillet, use it! Once you have your skillet, bring it over a moderate temperature and heat for several minutes without anything in it. Once hot, add in the steak and sear both sides for about three minutes. If you like your steak cooked past medium-rare, leave it on longer. When the steak is cooked to your liking, remove it from the pan and set to the side.
3. Now that your steak is cooked through, it is time to make the garlic butter. To accomplish this, you will want to lower the heat in your skillet and begin melting your butter. Once the butter has been liquified, you will next add in the garlic and cook for an additional minute. When the garlic turns a golden color, take the pan away from the heat.
4. The next step will be slicing up your steak. Once it is complete, carefully drizzle your butter sauce over the top until the steak becomes completely coated. As a final touch, garnish with some fresh parsley and enjoy your dinner.

NUTRITION: Calories: 190 Cal Fat: 23 g Carbs: 5 g Protein: 25 g Fiber: 3 g

17. Baked Lemon Salmon

Preparation Time:	10'		Servings:	4

	Cooking Time:	20'	

Ingredients

- 4 pieces of salmon
- A dash salt
- 2 tbsp. of lemon Juice
- 1 lemon
- 2 tbsps. of grass-fed Butter
- A dash pepper

Directions

1. If you enjoy your fresh seafood, this lemon salmon fillet is going to blow your mind. The lemon offers a refreshing twist to the fish and goes perfect with a side of cauliflower or broccoli. To start this recipe off, you will first want to go ahead and prep the stove to 400. As it heats up, get out your baking sheet and line it.
2. When you are set to cook the fish, you will first want to run it under water before patting it down with some paper towels. Once this has been done, place the fish with the skin side facing down.
3. Next, you will melt your butter and carefully spoon it over each piece of fish. With the butter in place, you can season with some pepper and salt according to your own taste.
4. Now that the fish has been seasoned, you will then want to pour your lemon juice over the top and place a slice of lemon on top of each salmon filet.
5. When you are ready to cook your meal, you are now going to pop the dish into the stove for fifteen minutes. By the end of this time, you will know that your fish is cooked through if you can flake it easily with a fork. If it is cooked through, take the dish out from the oven and allow it to chill for several minutes.
6. Finally, serve the fish with your favorite keto-friendly side, and enjoy your meal.

Nutrition: Calories: 150 Cal Fat: 20 g Carbs: 6 g Protein: 4 g Fiber: 1.6 g

18. One Sheet Fajitas

Preparation Time: 5'

Servings: 4

Cooking Time: 20'

Ingredients

- 1 lb. chicken breast
- 2 tbsps. fajita seasoning
- .25 cup of cilantro
- 1 sliced onion
- 1 slice red bell pepper
- 1 sliced green bell pepper
- 3 tbsps. of olive oil
- A dash salt
- 2 tbsps. of lime juice

Directions

1. What is better than fajitas for dinner? Fajitas that you can make using one pan! This recipe is easy to make and easy to enjoy. To begin, you will want to go ahead and prep the oven to 400. As this warms up, you can also get out the one baking sheet it is going to take for this recipe.
2. When you are all set, you will want to throw all of the ingredients from above into a mixing bowl and season with the pepper, salt, and the lime juice. Once this is set, spread the items across your baking sheet as evenly as possible.
3. Now that your sheet is set, you are going to pop it into the stove for twenty minutes. By the end of this time, the chicken should be cooked through. If you like everything a little crispy, you can go ahead and broil the ingredients for an additional two minutes.
4. When your meal is set, take it out from the stove and allow it to chill for two minutes. As a final touch, season with some fresh cilantro and enjoy your keto-friendly fajitas!

Nutrition: Calories: 158 Cal Fat: 19 g Carbs: 5 g Protein: 7g Fiber: 5 g

19. Balsamic Chicken

| PREPARATION TIME: | 10' | | SERVINGS: | 4 |

| COOKING TIME: | 50' |

Ingredients

- 4 pieces of chicken breast
- 2 tbsps. Of grass-fed butter
- A dash salt
- 4 roasted garlic cloves
- 2 cup sliced of mushrooms
- 1 tbsp. thyme

- 1 tbsp. chives
- 1 tbsp. red pepper flakes
- .25 cup of balsamic vinegar
- .50 cup of water
- .25 cup chopped onions

Directions

1. While following the Ketogenic Diet, it is a good idea always to have chicken on hand. This is a very versatile item and can offer a pack of protein as long as it is paired with the proper fats to balance out your diet. While this recipe does take a bit longer, the flavor will be worth the wait. You can begin this recipe by prepping the stove to 350 and getting out your baking sheet.
2. As the stove warms up, you will want to take out your skillet and begin heating the butter in it. Once the butter is melted, add in the chicken pieces and season with your pepper and salt. When the meat is seasoned to your liking, grill each side of the chicken for three or four minutes. Once the chicken is cooked through, place it onto your baking sheet, and cook in your heated stove for an additional twenty-five minutes.
3. As the chicken cooks, you will want to melt some more butter in your heated pan. Once melted, add in your mushrooms and onions. You will want to sauté these items for a minute before adding in the roasted garlic, thyme, red pepper flakes, and the balsamic vinegar. After these ingredients have cooked for a minute, pour in the water and stir until the liquid begins to reduce.
4. Finally, you are going to pour the mixture over your chicken and serve the dish hot. If you would like, you can serve with fresh parsley or chopped chives for some nice additional flavors.

NUTRITION: Calories: 168 Cal Fat: 4 g Carbs: 4 g Protein: 30 g Fiber: 3 g

20. Pesto Chicken Salad

Preparation Time: 4'

Servings: 4

Cooking Time: 20'

Ingredients

- 4 pieces' chicken breast
- .50 cup of pesto
- 1 cup cherry tomatoes
- 3 cups of spinach
- A dash salt
- 3 tbsps. of olive oil

Directions

1. For another alternative for plain old, baked chicken, you will want to consider this delicious Pesto chicken salad! To start off, you are going to want to go ahead and prep the stove to 350. As this warms up, place your chicken pieces onto a baking plate and coat with the pepper, salt, and olive oil. When this is done, pop the dish into the oven for forty minutes.
2. When the chicken is cooked through and no longer pink on the inside, you will now take it away from the oven and cool slightly before handling.
3. Once you can handle the chick, you will want to toss it into a bowl along with the pesto and your sliced tomatoes. When the ingredients are mended to your liking, place over a bowl of fresh spinach and enjoy your salad.

Nutrition: Calories: 188 Cal Fat: 19 g Carbs: 5 g Protein: 20 g Fiber: 3 g

21. Fresh Summer Salad

Preparation Time: 3'

Servings: 4

Cooking Time: 10'

Ingredients

- 2 tbsps. of olive oil
- 1 tbsp. of thyme
- 1 tbsp. oreano
- .25 cup of ricotta cheese
- 1 leaf, chopped basil
- 1 tbsp. of balsamic vinegar
- 1 sliced cucumber
- 3 sliced tomatoes
- 5 sliced radishes
- 1 sliced onion

Directions

1. Don't be fooled by the name; this salad can be enjoyed at any time of the year! If you are looking for a meatless dish, this is the perfect recipe for you! The first step you will want to take for this recipe will be making your ricotta cheese. You can complete this in a small bowl by mending the thyme, oregano, basil in with the ricotta cheese.
2. Next, you will be making your own dressing! For this task, all you have to do is whisk your vinegar and olive oil together. Once this is complete, season however you would like.
3. Finally, take some time to slice and dice the vegetables according to the directions above. When your veggies are all set, you will want to assemble them in your serving dishes and pour the dressing generously over the top. As a final touch, dollop your ricotta cheese over your salad, and then your salad will be ready for serving.

Nutrition: Calories: 158 Cal Fat: 19 g Carbs: 4 g Protein: 16 g Fiber: 2 g

22. Keto Taco Salad

Preparation Time: 5'	**Servings:** 4

Cooking Time: 20'

Ingredients

- 1 lb. ground beef
- 3 tbsp. of olive oil
- A dash pepper
- 1 tbsp. onion powder
- 1 tbsp. cumin
- 1 tbsp. minced garlic clove
- 1 chopped tomato
- .50 cup of sour cream
- .50 cup of black olives
- .25 cup of cheddar cheese
- 2 tbsps. cilantro
- 1 chopped green pepper

Directions

1. With taco salad, you will be able to enjoy everything that you love about tacos with a lot fewer carbohydrates! Whether you prepare this for taco Tuesday or a quick lunch, it is sure to be a crowd-pleaser!
2. Start this recipe off by taking out your grilling pan and place it over a moderate temperature. As it warms up, you can add in the olive oil and let that sizzle. When you are set, add in the green pepper, spices, and ground beef. You can also use ground turkey in this recipe if that is more your style. Go ahead and cook these ingredients together for ten minutes or so.
3. When you are all set, place some mixed greens into a bowl and cover with the meat mixture you just created. If you would like some extra flavor, sprinkle some cheddar cheese over the top along with some sour cream.

Nutrition: Calories: 138 Cal Fat: 27 g Carbs: 7 g Protein: 18 g Fiber: 5 g

23. Mixed Vegetable Tuna Salad

| PREPARATION TIME: | 10′ | SERVINGS: | 4 |

COOKING TIME: 0′

Ingredients

- 1 can canned tuna
- 2 tbsps. of olive oil
- .25 cup of parsley
- 1 roasted & chopped red pepper
- .50 cup diced of artichoke hearts
- .25 cup of black olives
- 2 tbsps. basil
- 2 tbsps. of lemon juice
- A dash pepper

Directions

1. When you are in a rush, you can't go wrong with tuna salad! To save yourself even more time, you can go ahead and prep this tuna salad at the beginning of the week so that all you will have to do is grab and go!
2. For this recipe, get out a mixing bowl and mend all of the items from the list above. Once combined, feel free to season with pepper and salt to your liking.
3. For serving purposes, this tuna salad can be enjoyed in a number of different ways. You can eat it right out of the bowl, scooped into a lettuce wrap, or served over a bed of salad!

NUTRITION: Calories: 256 Cal Fat: 16 g Carbs: 7 g Protein: 18 g Fiber: 3 g

24. Sausage and Cheese Puffs

Preparation Time: 5'	**Servings:** 4
Cooking Time: 30'	

Ingredients

- 4tbsps. melted butter
- 2 cup cheddar cheese
- 1 lb. sausage
- 4 eggs
- .25 tbsp. of garlic powder
- .25 tbsp. of baking powder
- .25 cup of coconut flour
- 3 tbsps. of sour cream
- A dash salt

Directions

1. For another quick and easy snack, you will want to try these little balls of heaven! They are soft, fluffy, and offer a good chunk of fat when you need it! This recipe can be used as a snack or can be an excellent addition to breakfast as well! To start off, you will want to prep the stove to 375. You can also get out a baking sheet; you are going to need it later.
2. Next, it is time to get out of the griddle! Go ahead and bring it over a moderate temperature. As it warms up, place your butter and let it melt. Once it is melted, add in your sausage and cook on both sides. Generally, this should only take three or four minutes. When it is cooked to your liking, take it out from the pan and set to the side.
3. Your next step will require a mixing bowl. Once you have your bowl, mend together the garlic, salt, sour cream, eggs, and four tablespoons of melted butter. When these are combined, add in the baking powder and coconut flour. Now that your dough is created, you will also want to fold in the cooked sausage and your shredded cheese.
4. Next, you will want to take your hands and make balls of batter. As you do this, line them up evenly across the surface of your baking sheet. When this is set, pop the dish into the stove for twenty minutes. By the end, the balls should be browned and cooked through.
5. If they are cooked to your liking, take the dish from the stove and chill slightly before digging into your snack.

Nutrition: Calories: 298 Cal Fat: 20 g Carbs: 4 g Protein: 8 g Fiber: 3 g

25. Frozen Berry Bites

Preparation Time: 15'

Servings: 4

Cooking Time: 3 hour

Ingredients

- 2 tbsps. of milk
- 2 cup full-fat yogurt
- .25 cup of blackberries
- .25 cup of raspberries
- 1 packet stevia

Directions

1. The fruit is generally left out of the Ketogenic Diet because it is high in sugar and carbs. However, sometimes it is nice to have as a treat! You will note that this recipe is slightly higher in carbohydrates, but as long as you count it with your macros, you can still enjoy some frozen berry bites in moderation!
2. To begin this recipe, you will first want to take some time to mash down the fruit into smaller pieces. When this is complete, you can add in your milk and yogurt. Once in place, combine everything together as well as possible so that the fruit is spread evenly.
3. When you are set, pour the mixture into an ice cube tray and pop into the freezer for about three hours. By the end, you can pop out the chunks, and your berry bites will be set for snack time.

Nutrition: Calories: 128 Cal Fat: 20 g Carbs: 5 g Protein: 8 g Fiber: 3 g

26. CREAM CHEESE AND HAM ROLLS

| PREPARATION TIME: | 5' | | SERVINGS: | 4 |

| COOKING TIME: | 0' |

INGREDIENTS

- 15 dill Pickles
- 1 package of cream cheese
- 15 slices of ham

DIRECTIONS

1. When you need a quick snack, this is the perfect recipe to whip together. Plus, finger foods can be a lot of fun if you are trying to get a child or friend to try out the Ketogenic Diet!
2. To make this quick and easy snack, you will first want to lay out each slice of ham in front of you. When this is done, carefully spread about a tablespoon of cream cheese across the surface. You will want to do this carefully because the ham can tear easily if the slices are not thick enough.
3. Finally, you are going to place one small pickle into the center and roll it up tightly. If needed, you can use a toothpick to keep your rolls in place.
4. When the step from above is complete, pop the dish into the fridge for at least two hours before serving.

NUTRITION: Calories: 148 Cal Fat: 30 g Carbs: 5 g Protein: 6 g Fiber: 4 g

27. Keto-friendly Crackers

Preparation Time:	10'		Servings:	25

	Cooking Time:	25'

Ingredients

- 2 cups of almond flour
- 2 eggs
- 8 tbsps. soft grass-fed butter
- A dash salt

Directions

1. While these crackers don't particularly offer a high amount of fat or protein, this recipe is great to have on hand. Crackers are versatile, whether you are looking for a snack or something on the side. You will find that many crackers in the market are filled with additives and high in carbs. To help keep them keto-friendly, you can make your own! To start out, prep the stove to 350 and get out your favorite baking sheet.
2. When you are set, take out a bowl and mend together the almond flour with the softened butter. For this step, it can be extremely helpful to have a hand mixer!
3. Once these two items are blended together, add in your eggs one at a time and punch some salt over the top. You will want to continue stirring these items until you get a perfectly smooth dough.
4. Next, you will want to place the dough in between two pieces of parchment paper and begin rolling out the dough onto your baking sheet. By doing this, you can make sure that the dough is flat and even. You will want to roll the dough out until it is about an eighth of an inch in thickness.
5. When you are done rolling the dough, use a pizza cutter to score your dough. You can make the crackers as big or as small as you would like! Once you have cut the dough up, pop the dish into the stove for fifteen minutes. By the end, the crackers should be golden.

Nutrition: Calories: 185 Cal Fat: 20 g Carbs: 6 g Protein: 9 g Fiber: 5 g

28. Keto Ice Cream

Preparation Time: 5'

Servings: 10

Cooking Time: 30'

Ingredients

- 2 egg yolks
- .50 cup of creamy peanut butter
- 2 cups heavy whipping cream
- 2 tbsps. cocoa powder, unsweetened
- .50 cup of erythritol

Directions

1. When you first start the Ketogenic Diet, you will quickly learn that all of your favorite foods are going to be high in carbs, high in added sugar, and filled with additives that are bad for your health. Luckily, you will be able to make a majority of your favorites all on your own! Here, we have simple chocolate and peanut butter ice cream that only requires five ingredients!
2. The first step of making your own ice cream will be taking out a mixing bowl and dissolving your cocoa powder. For this, you will only need about two tablespoons of water. When this is set, place it into a food processor with the rest of the ingredients and mend everything together for a few seconds.
3. When this is set, you are going to pour the mixture into a bowl and freeze for around three hours. After this, you will have delicious ice cream that is still keto-friendly! If you have an ice cream maker, you can also pour the mixture into here and have ice cream almost in an instant!

Nutrition: Calories: 148 Cal Fat: 20 g Carbs: 4 g Protein: 8 g Fiber: 3 g

29. Cheesecake Fat Bombs

PREPARATION TIME: 5'

SERVINGS: 15

COOKING TIME: 30'

INGREDIENTS

- .25 cup fresh raspberries
- 1 package cream cheese
- 2 tbsps. stevia
- 3 tbsps. of grass-fed butter
- 1 tbsp. of vanilla extract

DIRECTIONS

1. If you are a fan of cheesecake, you are going to love this recipe absolutely. By making these fat bombs, it is a great way to eat your cheesecake guilt-free because it is keto-friendly! Though it is delicious, remember to keep your dessert in moderation! Calories still count as calories, and there is such thing as too much fat on the Ketogenic Diet. You have to find the balance while still enjoying your treats.
2. To start this recipe, you will want to take some time to mash your raspberries down into smaller bits. Once the raspberry has been smashed, add in the cream cheese and the butter. To make this easier, you can leave the cream cheese and butter out at room temperature for around an hour or so.
3. Now that you have your mixture take your hands to create balls from the dough and place it into your freezer for thirty minutes. At the end of this time, your fat bombs will be solid and set for dessert.

NUTRITION: Calories: 125 Cal Fat: 10 g Carbs: 1 g Protein: 8 g Fiber: 3 g

30. Lemon Bars

Preparation Time: 10'	**Servings:** 8
Cooking Time: 60'	

Ingredients

- 2 cups of almond flour
- 2 lemons
- 3 eggs
- 1 cup of erythritol
- 25 cup of butter

Directions

1. Not everyone is a chocolate lover, and that is okay to admit! These lemon bars are dense and fluffy. If you need something to bring to a party, this is the perfect recipe to try out! You don't have to be following a Ketogenic Diet to enjoy this one.
2. You will want to start this recipe off by prepping the stove to 350. As the stove heats up, line your baking dish with some paper and begin mixing together the almond flour with the erythritol. For a touch more of flavor, feel free to add a pinch of salt.
3. When you are set, pour the mixture into your baking dish and pop it into the stove for twenty minutes. By the end of this time, the bars should be set and can be taken out of the oven.
4. Next, it is time to make the lemon zest for your bars! In a bowl, you will want to juice the two lemons and add the zest from one. When these are set, mix in your eggs along with a cup of erythritol and another cup of your almond flour. Once this step is complete, pour it onto the crust and pop the dish back into the stove for an additional twenty-five minutes.
5. When your bars are cooked to your liking, take the dish from the oven and allow it to chill for ten minutes before slicing the bars up. For a finishing touch, sprinkle some more erythritol over the top and even decorate with a slice of lemon!

Nutrition: Calories: 168 Cal Fat: 20 g Carbs: 5 g Protein: 8 g Fiber: 3 g

31. Keto Baked Salmon with Lemon and Butter

| PREPARATION TIME: | 10' | | SERVINGS: | 3 |

| COOKING TIME: | 30' |

Ingredients

- 1 pound salmon
- 1 lemon
- 3 ozs. butter
- 1 tablespoon olive oil
- Ground black pepper and sea salt to taste

Directions

1. Grease a large-sized baking dish with the olive oil and preheat your oven to 400°F.
2. Place the salmon on the baking dish, preferably skin-side down. Generously season with pepper and salt to taste.
3. Thinly slice the lemon and place the slices over the salmon. Cover the fish with ½ of the butter, preferably in very thin slices.
4. Bake until the salmon flakes easily with a fork and is opaque, for 25 to 30 minutes, on the middle rack.
5. Now, over moderate heat in a small saucepan; heat the remaining butter until it begins to bubble. Immediately remove the pan from heat; set aside and let cool a bit. Gently add in some of the freshly squeezed lemon juice.
6. Serve the cooked fish with some of the prepared lemon butter and enjoy it.

NUTRITION: Calories: 298 Cal Fat: 20 g Carbs: 4 g Protein: 8 g Fiber: 3 g

32. Ketogenic Spicy Oyster

Preparation Time: 10'

Servings: 2

Cooking Time: 5'

Ingredients

- 12 oysters shucked
- 1 tablespoon olive oil
- 7-8 basil leaves, fresh
- 1 tablespoon garlic chili paste
- 1/8 teaspoon salt

Directions

1. Combine olive oil with garlic chili paste and salt in a medium-size mixing bowl; mix well.
2. Add oysters into the prepared sauce; turning them several times until thoroughly coated.
3. Create a bed for the oysters to cook by spreading the basil leaves out on an oven-safe dish.
4. Transfer the oysters and sauce over the bed of basil leaves; spreading them in a single layer on the dish.
5. Turn on the broiler over high heat.
6. Place the dish on the top rack (approximately a few inches away from the broiler) and broil for a few minutes.
7. Once done, immediately remove them from the oven. Serve hot and enjoy.

Nutrition: Calories: 158 Cal Fat: 16 g Carbs: 2 g Protein: 6 g Fiber: 8 g

33. GARLIC LIME MAHI-MAHI

PREPARATION TIME: 45'

SERVINGS: 4

COOKING TIME: 10'

INGREDIENTS

- 4 Mahi-Mahi filets (approximately 1 to 1 ¼ pounds)
- Zest and juice of 1 large lime, fresh
- ¼ cup avocado oil
- 3 cloves garlic, minced
- 1/8 teaspoon each of ground black pepper and fine grain sea salt

DIRECTIONS

1. For Marinade: Thoroughly combine the entire ingredients (except the filets) together in a small-sized mixing bowl. Pour the mixture on top of the filets in a large zip-lock bag or large shallow dish. Let marinate for 30 minutes, at room temperature.
2. Pour the marinade into a large sauté pan (preferably with a cover) and heat it over medium heat. Once hot; carefully add the filets into the hot pan; cover and cook the filets for a couple of minutes, until cooked through.
3. Immediately remove the sauté pan from heat; set aside and let rest for 5 minutes, covered. Serve warm and enjoy.

NUTRITION: Calories: 153 Cal Fat: 13 g Carbs: 5 g Protein: 2 g Fiber: 3 g

34. Fish and Leek Sauté

Preparation Time: 15'	**Servings:** 2
Cooking Time: 10'	

Ingredients

- 1 leek, chopped
- 2 trout fillets, diced (approximately 8 ozs.)
- 1 tablespoon tamari soy sauce
- 1 teaspoon ginger, grated
- 1 tablespoon avocado oil
- Salt to taste

Directions

1. Over moderate heat in a large skillet; heat the avocado oil until hot. Once done; add and sauté the chopped leek for a few minutes, until turn soften.
2. Immediately add the diced trout with grated ginger, tamari sauce, and salt to taste.
3. Continue to sauté the trout until it's not translucent anymore and cooked through.
4. Serve immediately and enjoy it.

Nutrition: Calories: 134 Cal Fat: 21 g Carbs: 4 g Protein: 8 g Fiber: 3 g

35. Smoked Salmon Salad

Preparation Time:	5'		Servings:	1

Cooking Time:	0'

Ingredients

- 2 ozs. smoked salmon
- 1 lemon slice
- 4 olives
- 1 teaspoon pink peppercorns, crushed lightly
- A handful of arugula salad leaves, fresh

Directions

1. Place the olives and salad leaves into a large plate or shallow bowl.
2. Arrange the smoked salmon over the salad.
3. Sprinkle the top of smoked salmon with lightly crushed pink peppercorns.
4. Garnish your salad with a lemon slice; serve immediately and enjoy.

Nutrition: Calories: 178 Cal Fat: 22 g Carbs: 4 g Protein: 7 g Fiber: 2 g

36. Keto Baked Salmon with Pesto

Preparation Time: 10'	**Servings:** 2
Cooking Time: 30'	

Ingredients

- 1 oz. green pesto
- ½ pound salmon
- Pepper and salt to taste

For Green sauce:
- ¼ cup Greek yogurt
- 1 oz. green pesto
- ¼ teaspoon garlic
- Pepper and salt to taste

Directions

1. Preheat your oven to 400°F.
2. Arrange the salmon in a well-greased baking dish, preferably skin-side down. Spread the pesto over the salmon and then, sprinkle with pepper and salt to taste.
3. Bake in the preheated oven until the salmon flakes easily with a fork, for 25 to 30 minutes.
4. In the meantime, stir the entire sauce ingredients together in a large bowl. Serve the cooked fish with some of the prepared sauce and enjoy it.

Nutrition: Calories: 158 Cal Fat: 18g Carbs: 6 g Protein: 5 g Fiber: 3 g

37. Roasted Salmon with Parmesan Dill Crust

Preparation Time:	10′		Servings:	2

Cooking Time:	10′

Ingredients

- ½ pound salmon; cut into pieces
- 1 tablespoon dill weed
- ¼ cup cottage cheese
- 1 tablespoon olive oil
- ¼ cup parmesan cheese, grated

Directions

1. Preheat your oven to 450°F.
2. Combine cottage cheese with parmesan cheese, olive oil, and dill in a large-sized mixing bowl; mix well.
3. Line a large-sized baking sheet with aluminum foil and then, arrange the salmon pieces on it.
4. Smear ½ of the cottage cheese mixture over the salmon.
5. Roast in the preheated oven until the fish flakes easily and the crust is brown, for 10 minutes.
6. Serve the cooked fish with the remaining prepared sauce and enjoy it.

Nutrition: Calories: 159 Cal Fat: 19 g Carbs: 6 g Protein: 4 g Fiber: 6 g

38. Keto Fried Salmon with Broccoli and Cheese

PREPARATION TIME: 15'	SERVINGS: 3

COOKING TIME: 25'

INGREDIENTS

- ¾ pound salmon; cut into pieces
- 3 tablespoons butter
- ½ pound broccoli; cut into small florets
- 2 ozs. cheddar cheese, grated
- Pepper and salt to taste
- 1 lime

DIRECTIONS

1. Preheat the oven to 400°F (200°C), preferably using the broiler setting.
2. Cut the broccoli into smaller florets and let simmer in lightly salted water for a couple of minutes. Make sure the broccoli maintains its chewy texture and delicate color.
3. Drain the broccoli and discard the boiling water. Set aside, uncovered, for a minute or two to allow the steam to evaporate.
4. Place the drained broccoli in a well-greased baking dish. Add butter and pepper to taste.
5. Sprinkle cheese on top of the broccoli and bake in the oven for 15-20 minutes or until the cheese turns a golden color.
6. In the meantime, season the salmon with salt and pepper and fry in plenty of butter, a few minutes on each side. The lime can be fried in the same pan or be served raw. This step can also be made on an outdoor grill.

NUTRITION: Calories: 328 Cal Fat: 27 g Carb: 7 g Protein: 5 g Fiber: 3 g

39. Keto Rib Eye Steak

| PREPARATION TIME: | 5' | | SERVINGS: | 2 |

| COOKING TIME: | 20' |

INGREDIENTS

- ½ pound grass-fed rib-eye steak, preferably 1" thick
- 1 teaspoon Adobo Seasoning
- 1 tablespoon extra-virgin olive oil
- Pepper and sea salt to taste

DIRECTIONS

1. Add steak in a large-sized mixing bowl and drizzle both sides with a small amount of olive oil. Dust the seasonings on both sides; rubbing the seasonings into the meat.
2. Let sit for a couple of minutes and heat up your grill in advance. Once hot; place the steaks over the grill, and cook until both sides are cooked through, for 15 to 20 minutes, flipping occasionally.

NUTRITION: Calories: 258 Cal Fat: 19 g Carbs: 5 g Protein: 8 g Fiber: 8 g

40. Bacon Bleu Zoodle Salad

Preparation Time:	5′		Servings:	2

	Cooking Time:	0′	

Ingredients

- 4 cups zucchini noodles
- ½ cup bacon, cooked and crumbled
- 1 cup fresh spinach, chopped
- 1/3 cup bleu cheese, crumbled
- Fresh cracked pepper, to taste

Directions

1. Toss the entire ingredients together in a large-sized mixing bowl. Serve immediately, and enjoy.

Nutrition: Calories: 268 Cal Fat: 18 g Carbs: 7 g Protein: 8 g Fiber: 3 g

41. Garlic Baked Butter Chicken

| PREPARATION TIME: | 10' | | SERVINGS: | 4 |

| COOKING TIME: | 40' |

INGREDIENTS

- 1 tablespoon rosemary leaves, fresh
- 3 chicken breasts, boneless, skinless (approximately 12 ozs.); washed and cleaned
- 1 stick butter (½ cup)
- ½ cup Italian cheese, low fat and shredded
- 6 garlic cloves, minced
- Fresh ground pepper and salt to taste

DIRECTIONS

1. Grease a large-sized baking dish lightly with a pat of butter, and preheat your oven to 375°F.
2. Season the chicken breasts with pepper and salt to taste; arrange them in the prepared baking dish, preferably in a single layer; set aside.
3. Now, over medium heat in a large skillet; heat the butter until melted, and then cook the garlic until lightly browned, for 4 to 5 minutes, stirring every now and then. Keep an eye on the garlic; don't burn it.
4. Add the rosemary; give everything a good stir; remove the skillet from heat.
5. Transfer the already prepared garlic butter over the meat.
6. Bake in the preheated oven for 30 minutes.
7. Sprinkle cheese on top and cook until the cheese is completely melted, for a couple of more minutes.
8. Remove from the oven and let stand for a couple of minutes. Transfer the cooked meat to large serving plates. Serve and enjoy.

NUTRITION: Calories: 178 Cal Fat: 18 g Carbs: 6 g Protein: 12 g Fiber: 3 g

42. Lemon Rosemary Chicken Thighs

Preparation Time: 10'	**Servings:** 4
Cooking Time: 45'	

Ingredients

- 4 chicken thighs
- 2 garlic cloves, roughly chopped
- 4 sprigs of Rosemary, fresh
- 1 lemon, medium
- 2 tablespoons butter
- Pepper, and salt to taste

Directions

1. Preheat your oven to 400F° in advance and heat up a cast-iron skillet over high heat as well.
2. Season both sides of the meat with pepper, and salt. When the skillet is hot; carefully place the coated thighs, preferably skin side down into the hot skillet and sear them for 4 to 5 minutes, until nicely brown.
3. Carefully flip and flavor the thighs with the lemon juice (only use ½ of the lemon). Quarter the leftover lemon halves and throw the pieces into the pan with the chicken.
4. Add the chopped garlic cloves together with some rosemary into the skillet.
5. Place the skillet inside the oven and bake for 30 minutes.
6. Remove the skillet from the oven. To add flavor, moisture, and more of crispiness; add a portion of butter over the chicken thighs. Bake for 10 more minutes.
7. Serve hot and enjoy.

Nutrition: Calories: 302 Cal Fat: 18 g Carbs: 5 g Protein: 8 g Fiber: 4 g

43. Coffee Butter Rubbed Tri-Tip Steak

PREPARATION TIME:	20'		SERVINGS:	2

COOKING TIME:	15'

INGREDIENTS

- 2 Tri-tip steaks, preferably ½ pound
- 1 package of coffee blocks
- ½ tablespoon garlic powder
- 1 teaspoon black pepper, coarse ground
- 2 tablespoons olive oil
- ½ tablespoon of sea salt

DIRECTIONS

1. Pound the meat using a mallet until tenderize; let the meat sit for 20 minutes at room temperature.
2. Combine everything together (except the steaks) in a large-sized mixing bowl.
3. Rub the sides, top, and bottom of the meat steaks entirely with the mixture.
4. Over medium-high heat in a large skillet; heat the olive oil until hot.
5. Carefully add the coated steaks into the hot oil and cook for 5 minutes.
6. Flip and cook the other side until cooked through, for 5 more minutes.
7. Remove the meat from the pan and let sit for a minute in its own juices.
8. Cut into slices against the grain. Serve warm and enjoy.

NUTRITION: Calories: 206 Cal Fat: 19 g Carbs: 5 g Protein:10 g Fiber: 3.2 g

44. KETO GROUND BEEF AND GREEN BEANS

PREPARATION TIME:	5'	SERVINGS:	2

COOKING TIME: 10'

INGREDIENTS

- 1 ½ oz. butter
- 8 ozs. green beans, fresh, rinsed, and trimmed
- 10 ozs. ground beef
- 1/4 cup Crème Fraiche or home-made mayonnaise, optional
- Pepper and salt to taste

DIRECTIONS

1. Over moderate heat in a large, frying pan; heat a generous dollop of butter until completely melted.
2. Increase the heat to high and immediately brown the ground beef until almost done, for 5 minutes. Sprinkle with pepper and salt to taste.
3. Decrease the heat to medium; add more of butter and continue to fry the beans in the same pan with the meat for 5 more minutes, stirring frequently.
4. Season the beans with pepper and salt as well. Serve with the leftover butter and add in the optional Crème Fraiche or mayonnaise, if desired.

NUTRITION: Calories: 238 Cal Fat: 15 g Carbs: 8 g Protein: 10 g Fiber: 4 g

45. Spicy Beef Meatballs

| PREPARATION TIME: | 10' | | SERVINGS: | 3 |

| COOKING TIME: | 10' |

INGREDIENTS

- 1 cup mozzarella or cheddar cheese; cut into 1x1 cm cubes
- 1 pound minced ground beef
- 1 teaspoon olive oil
- 3 tablespoons parmesan cheese
- 1 teaspoon garlic powder
- ½ teaspoon each of pepper, and salt

DIRECTIONS

1. Thoroughly combine the ground beef with the entire dry ingredients; mix well.
2. Wrap the cheese cubes into the mince; forming 9 meatballs from the prepared mixture.
3. Pan-fry the formed meatballs until cooked through, covered (uncover and stirring frequently).

NUTRITION: Calories: 358 Cal Fat: 19 g Carbs: 4 g Protein: 18 g Fiber: 5 g

46. Chilled Cucumber Soup

Preparation Time:	15'		Servings:	2

Cooking Time:	0'

Ingredients

- 1 cup English cucumber, peeled and chopped
- 1 scallion, chopped
- 2 tablespoons fresh parsley leaves
- 2 tablespoons fresh basil leaves
- ¼ teaspoon fresh lime zest, grated freshly
- 1 cup unsweetened coconut milk
- ¼ cup of water
- ½ tablespoon fresh lime juice
- Salt and ground black pepper, as required

Directions

1. Add all the ingredients in a high-speed blender and pulse on high speed until smooth.
2. Transfer the soup into a large serving bowl.
3. Cover the bowl of soup and place in the refrigerator to chill for about 6 hours.
4. Serve chilled.

Nutrition: Calories: 198 Cal Fat: 10 g Carbs: 7 g Protein: 9 g Fiber: 5 g

47. Creamy Mushroom Soup

Preparation Time: 15'

Servings: 4

Cooking Time: 20'

Ingredients

- 3 tablespoons unsalted butter
- 1 scallion, sliced
- 1 large garlic clove, crushed
- 5 cups fresh button mushrooms, sliced
- 2 cups homemade vegetable broth
- Salt and ground black pepper, as required
- 1 cup heavy cream

Directions

1. In a large soup pan, melt the butter over medium heat and sauté the scallion and garlic for about 2–3 minutes.
2. Add the mushrooms cook fry for about 5–6 minutes, stirring frequently.
3. Stir in the broth and bring to a boil.
4. Cook for about 5 minutes.
5. Remove from the heat and with a stick blender, blend the soup until smooth.
6. Return the pan over medium heat.
7. Stir in the cream, salt, and black pepper and cook for about 2–3 minutes, stirring continuously.
8. Remove from the heat and serve hot

Nutrition: Calories: 195 Cal Fat: 17 g Carbs: 8 g Protein: 2 g Fiber: 5 g

48. Broccoli Soup

Preparation Time: 10'	**Servings:** 2

Cooking Time: 15'

Ingredients

- 5 cups homemade chicken broth
- 20 ounces' small broccoli florets
- 12 ounces' cheddar cheese, cubed
- Salt and ground black pepper, as required
- 1 cup heavy cream

Directions

1. In a large soup pan, add the broth and broccoli over medium-high heat and bring to a boil.
2. Reduce the heat to low and simmer, covered for about 5–7 minutes.
3. Stir in the cheese and cook for about 2–3 minutes, stirring continuously.
4. Stir in the salt, black pepper, and cream, and cook for about 2 minutes.
5. Serve hot.

Nutrition: Calories: 170 Cal Fat: 14 g Carbs: 2 g Protein:6 g Fiber: 3 g

49. MEATBALLS SOUP

PREPARATION TIME: 20'

COOKING TIME: 25'

SERVINGS: 6

INGREDIENTS

- 1 pound lean ground turkey
- 1 garlic clove, minced
- 1 organic egg, beaten
- ¼ cup Parmesan cheese, grated
- Salt and ground black pepper, as required

Soup
- 1 tablespoon olive oil
- 1 small yellow onion, finely chopped
- 1 garlic clove, minced
- 6 cups homemade chicken broth
- 7 cups fresh spinach, chopped
- Salt and ground black pepper, as required

DIRECTIONS

For meatballs: In a bowl, add all ingredients and mix until well combined.

1. Make equal sized small balls from the mixture.
2. In a large soup pan, heat oil over medium heat and sauté onion for about 5–6 minutes.
3. Add the garlic and sauté for about 1 minute.
4. Add in the broth and bring to a boil.
5. Carefully, place the balls in the pan and bring to a boil.
6. Reduce the heat to low and cook for about 10 minutes.
7. Stir in the kale and bring the soup to a gentle simmer.
8. Simmer for about 2–3 minutes.
9. Season the soup with the salt and black pepper and serve hot.:

NUTRITION: Calories: 198 Cal Fat: 17 g Carbs: 9 g Protein: 7 g Fiber: 4 g

50. SHRIMP WITH ASPARAGUS

PREPARATION TIME: 15'

SERVINGS: 4

COOKING TIME: 10'

INGREDIENTS

- 2 tablespoons butter
- 1 pound asparagus, trimmed
- 1 pound shrimp, peeled and deveined
- 4 garlic cloves, minced
- 2 tablespoons fresh lemon juice
- 1/3 cup homemade chicken broth

DIRECTIONS

1. Melt butter in a large wok over medium-high heat.
2. Add all the ingredients except broth and cook for about 2 minutes, without stirring.
3. Stir the mixture and cook for about 3–4 minutes, stirring occasionally.
4. Stir in the broth and cook for about 2–4 more minutes.
5. Serve hot.

NUTRITION: Calories: 218 Cal Fat: 17 g Carbs: 8 g Protein: 9 g Fiber: 4 g

51. Shrimp Curry

Preparation Time: 15'

Servings: 4

Cooking Time: 21'

Ingredients

- 2 tablespoons coconut oil
- ½ of yellow onion, minced
- 2 garlic cloves, minced
- 1 teaspoon ground turmeric
- 1 teaspoon ground cumin
- 1 teaspoon paprika
- 1 (14-ounce) can unsweetened coconut milk
- 1 large tomato, chopped finely
- Salt, as required
- 1 pound shrimp, peeled and deveined
- 2 tablespoons fresh cilantro, chopped

Directions

1. Melt coconut oil in a large wok over medium heat and sauté the onion for about 5 minutes.
2. Add the garlic, and spices, and sauté for about 1 minute.
3. Add the coconut milk, tomato, and salt, and bring to a gentle boil.
4. Lower the heat to low and simmer for about 10 minutes, stirring occasionally.
5. Stir in the shrimp and cilantro and simmer for about 4–5 minutes.
6. Remove the wok from heat and serve hot.

Nutrition: Calories: 168 Cal Fat: 15g Carbs: 5 g Protein: 9 g Fiber: 7 g

52. SEAFOOD STEW

PREPARATION TIME: 20'

SERVINGS: 8

COOKING TIME: 30'

INGREDIENTS

- 2 tablespoons butter
- 1 medium yellow onion, chopped
- 2 garlic cloves, minced
- 1 Serrano pepper, chopped
- ¼ teaspoon red pepper flakes, crushed
- ½ pound fresh tomatoes, chopped
- 1½ cups homemade fish broth
- 1 pound red snapper fillets, cubed
- ½ pound shrimp, peeled and deveined
- ¼ pound fresh squid, cleaned and cut into rings
- ¼ pound bay scallops
- ¼ pound mussels
- 2 tablespoons fresh lime juice
- ½ cup fresh basil, chopped

DIRECTIONS

1. In a large soup pan, melt butter over medium heat and sauté the onion for about 5–6 minutes.
2. Add the garlic, Serrano pepper, and red pepper flakes, and sauté for about 1 minute.
3. Add tomatoes and broth and bring to a gentle simmer.
4. Reduce the heat and cook for about 10 minutes.
5. Add the tilapia and cook for about 2 minutes.
6. Stir in the remaining seafood and cook for about 6–8 minutes.
7. Stir in the lemon juice, basil, salt, and black pepper, and remove from heat.
8. Serve hot.

NUTRITION: Calories: 199 Cal Fat: 12.1 g Carbs: 7.5 g Protein: 8 g Fiber: 3 g

53. Tomato & Mozzarella Salad

PREPARATION TIME:	15'	SERVINGS:	8

COOKING TIME:	15'

INGREDIENTS

- 4 cups cherry tomatoes, halved
- 1½ pounds mozzarella cheese, cubed
- ¼ cup fresh basil leaves, chopped
- ¼ cup olive oil
- 2 tablespoons fresh lemon juice
- 1 teaspoon fresh oregano, minced
- 1 teaspoon fresh parsley, minced
- 2–4 drops liquid stevia
- Salt and ground black pepper, as required

DIRECTIONS

1. In a salad bowl, mix together tomatoes, mozzarella, and basil.
2. In a small bowl, add remaining ingredients and beat until well combined.
3. Place dressing over salad and toss to coat well.
4. Serve immediately.

NUTRITION: Calories: 310 Cal Fat: 18 g Carbs: 7 g Protein: 8 g Fiber: 3 g

54. Cucumber & Tomato Salad

Preparation Time: 15'

Servings: 8

Cooking Time: 15'

Ingredients

Salad:
- 3 large English cucumbers, thinly sliced
- 2 cups tomatoes, chopped
- 6 cups lettuce, torn

Dressing:
- 4 tablespoons olive oil
- 2 tablespoons balsamic vinegar
- 1 tablespoon fresh lemon juice
- Salt and ground black pepper, as required

Directions

1. For salad: In a large bowl, add the cucumbers, onion, cucumbers, and mix.
2. For dressing: In a small bowl, add all the ingredients and beat until well combined.
3. Place the dressing over the salad and toss to coat well.
4. Serve immediately.

Nutrition: Calories: 268 Cal Fat: 18 g Carbs: 7 g Protein: 8 g Fiber: 3 g

55. Chicken & Broccoli Casserole

PREPARATION TIME: 15'

SERVINGS: 6

COOKING TIME: 35'

Ingredients

- 2 tablespoons butter
- ¼ cup cooked bacon, crumbled
- 2½ cups cheddar cheese, shredded and divided
- 4 ounces' cream cheese, softened
- ¼ cup heavy whipping cream
- ½ pack ranch seasoning mix
- 2/3 cup homemade chicken broth
- 1½ cups small broccoli florets
- 2 cups cooked grass-fed chicken breast, shredded

Directions

1. Preheat your oven to 350ºF.
2. Arrange a rack in the upper portion of the oven.
3. For chicken mixture: In a large wok, melt the butter over low heat.
4. Add the bacon, ½ cup of cheddar cheese, cream cheese, heavy whipping cream, ranch seasoning, and broth, and with a wire whisk, beat until well combined.
5. Cook for about 5 minutes, stirring frequently.
6. Meanwhile, in a microwave-safe dish, place the broccoli and microwave until desired tenderness is achieved.
7. In the wok, add the chicken and broccoli and mix until well combined.
8. Remove from the heat and transfer the mixture into a casserole dish.
9. Top the chicken mixture with the remaining cheddar cheese.
10. Bake for about 25 minutes.
11. Now, set the oven to broiler.
12. Broil the chicken mixture for about 2–3 minutes or until cheese is bubbly.
13. Serve hot.

NUTRITION: Calories: 168 Cal Fat: 19 g Carbs: 8 g Protein: 10 g Fiber: 5 g

56. Turkey Chili

Preparation Time:	15'	**Servings:**	8

Cooking Time: 120'

Ingredients

- 2 tablespoons olive oil
- 1 small yellow onion, chopped
- 1 green bell pepper, seeded and chopped
- 4 garlic cloves, minced
- 1 jalapeño pepper, chopped
- 1 teaspoon dried thyme, crushed
- 2 tablespoons red chili powder
- 1 tablespoon ground cumin
- 2 pounds lean ground turkey
- 2 cups fresh tomatoes, chopped finely
- 2 ounces' sugar-free tomato paste
- 2 cups homemade chicken broth
- 1 cup of water
- Salt and ground black pepper, as required
- 1 cup cheddar cheese, shredded

Directions

1. In a large Dutch oven, heat oil over medium heat and sauté the onion and bell pepper for about 5–7 minutes.
2. Add the garlic, jalapeño pepper, thyme, and spices and sauté for about 1 minute.
3. Add the turkey and cook for about 4–5 minutes.
4. Stir in the tomatoes, tomato paste, and cacao powder, and cook for about 2 minutes.
5. Add in the broth and water and bring to a boil.
6. Now, reduce the heat to low and simmer, covered for about 2 hours.
7. Add in salt and black pepper and remove from the heat.
8. Top with cheddar cheese and serve hot.

Nutrition: Calories: 308 Cal Fat: 20 g Carbs: 10 g Protein: 8 g Fiber: 3 g

57. Beef Curry

Preparation Time:	10'	**Servings:**	8

Cooking Time: 205'

Ingredients

- 2 tablespoons butter
- 2 tomatoes, chopped finely
- 2 tablespoons curry powder
- 2½ cups unsweetened coconut milk
- ½ cup homemade chicken broth
- 2½ pounds grass-fed beef chuck roast, cubed into 1-inch size
- Salt and ground black pepper, as required
- ¼ cup fresh cilantro, chopped

Directions

1. Melt butter in a big pan over low heat and cook the tomatoes and curry powder for about 3–4 minutes, crushing the tomatoes with the back of spoon.
2. Stir in the coconut milk, and broth, and bring to a gentle simmer, stirring occasionally.
3. Simmer for about 4–5 minutes.
4. Stir in beef and bring to a boil over medium heat.
5. Adjust the heat to low and cook, covered for about 2½ hours, stirring occasionally
6. Remove from heat and with a slotted spoon, transfer the beef into a bowl.
7. Set the pan of curry aside for about 10 minutes.
8. With a slotted spoon, remove the fats from top of curry.
9. Return the pan over medium heat.
10. Stir in the cooked beef and bring to a gentle simmer.
11. Adjust the heat to low and cook, uncovered for about 30 minutes, or until desired thickness.
12. Stir in salt and black pepper and remove from the heat.
13. Garnish with fresh cilantro and serve hot.

Nutrition: Calories: 360 Cal Fat: 25 g Carbs: 3 g Protein: 18 g Fiber: 3 g

58. Shepherd's Pie

Preparation Time: 20'

Servings: 6

Cooking Time: 50'

Ingredients

- ¼ cup olive oil
- 1 pound grass-fed ground beef
- ½ cup celery, chopped
- ¼ cup yellow onion, chopped
- 3 garlic cloves, minced
- 1 cup tomatoes, chopped
- 2 (12-ounce) packages riced cauliflower, cooked and well-drained
- 1 cup cheddar cheese, shredded

Directions

1. Preheat your oven to 350°F.
2. Heat oil in a large nonstick wok over medium heat and cook the ground beef, celery, onions, and garlic for about 8–10 minutes.
3. Remove from the heat and drain the excess grease.
4. Immediately stir in the tomatoes.
5. Transfer mixture into a 10x7-inch casserole dish evenly.
6. In a food processor, add the cauliflower, cheeses, cream, and thyme, and pulse until a mashed potatoes-like mixture is formed.
7. Spread the cauliflower mixture over the meat in the casserole dish evenly.
8. Bake for about 35–40 minutes.
9. Remove casserole dish from oven and let it cool slightly before serving.
10. Cut into desired sized pieces and serve.

Nutrition: Calories: 404 Cal Fat: 19 g Carbs: 10 g Protein: 19 g Fiber:5 g

59. Pork with Veggies

Preparation Time: 15'

Servings: 5

Cooking Time: 15'

Ingredients

- 1 quid pork loin, cut into thin strips
- 2 tablespoons olive oil, divided
- 1 teaspoon garlic, minced
- 1 teaspoon fresh ginger, minced
- 2 tablespoons low-sodium soy sauce
- 1 tablespoon fresh lemon juice
- 1 teaspoon sesame oil
- 1 tablespoon granulated erythritol
- 1 teaspoon arrowroot star
- 10 ounces' broccoli florets
- 1 carrot, peeled and sliced
- 1 big red bell pepper, seeded and cut into strips
- 2 scallions, cut into 2-inch pieces

Directions

1. In a bowl, mix well pork strips, ½ tablespoon of olive oil, garlic, and ginger.
2. For the sauce: Add the soy sauce, lemon juice, sesame oil, Swerve, and arrowroot starch in a small bowl and mix well.
3. Heat the remaining olive oil in a big nonstick wok over high heat and sear the pork strips for about 3–4 minutes or until cooked through.
4. With a slotted spoon, transfer the pork into a bowl.
5. In the same wok, add the carrot and cook for about 2–3 minutes.
6. Add the broccoli, bell pepper, and scallion, and cook, covered for about 1–2 minutes.
7. Stir the cooked pork, sauce, and stir fry, and cook for about 3–5 minutes or until desired doneness, stirring occasionally.
8. Remove from the heat and serve.

Nutrition: Calories: 268 Cal Fat: 18 g Carbs: 7 g Protein: 8 g Fiber: 3 g

60. Pork Taco Bake

Preparation Time: 15'	**Servings:** 6
Cooking Time: 60'	

Ingredients

Crust
- 3 organic eggs
- 4 ounces' cream cheese, softened
- ½ teaspoon taco seasoning
- 1/3 cup heavy cream
- 8 ounces' cheddar cheese, shredded

Topping:
- 1 pound lean ground pork
- 4 ounces canned chopped green chilies
- ¼ cup sugar-free tomato sauce
- 3 teaspoons taco seasoning
- 8 ounces' cheddar cheese, shredded
- ¼ cup fresh basil leaves

Directions

1. Preheat your oven to 375°F.
2. Lightly grease a 13x9-inch baking dish.
3. For crust: In a bowl, add the eggs and cream cheese, and beat until well combined and smooth.
4. Add the taco seasoning and heavy cream, and mix well.
5. Place cheddar cheese evenly in the bottom of prepared baking dish.
6. Spread cream cheese mixture evenly over cheese.
7. Bake for about 25–30 minutes.
8. Remove baking dish from the oven and set aside for about 5 minutes.
9. Meanwhile, for the topping: Heat a large nonstick wok over medium-high heat and cook the pork for about 8–10 minutes.
10. Drain the excess grease from wok.
11. Stir in the green chilies, tomato sauce, and taco seasoning, and remove from the heat.
12. Place the pork mixture evenly over crust and sprinkle with cheese.
13. Bake for about 18–20 minutes or until bubbly.
14. Remove from the oven and set aside for about 5 minutes.
15. Cut into desired size slices and serve with the garnishing of basil leaves.

Nutrition: Calories: 198 Cal Fat: 12 g Carbs: 8 g Protein: 19 g Fiber: 3 g

61. Shrimp Lettuce Wraps

Preparation Time: 20'

Servings: 6

Cooking Time: 4'

Ingredients

Shrimp:
- 1 teaspoon olive oil
- 2 pounds' shrimp, peeled, deveined, and chopped
- ½ teaspoon ground cumin
- 1 teaspoon red chili powder
- Salt and ground black pepper, to taste

Wraps:
- 1 cup tomato, chopped finely
- ½ cup onion, chopped
- 2 tablespoons fresh parsley, chopped
- 12 butter lettuce leaves

Directions

1. For shrimp: In a large wok, heat the oil over medium heat and cook the shrimp, spices, salt, and black pepper for about 3–4 minutes.
2. Remove the wok from the heat and set aside to cool slightly.
3. Meanwhile, in a bowl, mix together tomato, onion, and parsley.
4. Arrange the lettuce leaves onto serving plates.
5. Divide the shrimp over lettuce leaves evenly.
6. Top with tomato mixture evenly and serve.

Nutrition: Calories: 199 Cal Fat: 18 g Carbs: 4 g Protein: 9 g Fiber: 5 g

62. CHICKEN STUFFED AVOCADO

PREPARATION TIME: 15'

SERVINGS: 2

COOKING TIME: 0'

INGREDIENTS

- 1 cup grass-fed cooked chicken, shredded
- 1 avocado, halved and pitted
- 1 tablespoon fresh lime juice
- ¼ cup yellow onion, chopped finely
- ¼ cup plain Greek yogurt
- 1 teaspoon Dijon mustard
- Pinch of cayenne pepper
- Salt and ground black pepper, to taste

DIRECTIONS

1. With a spoon, scoop out the flesh from the middle of each avocado half and transfer into a bowl.
2. Add the lime juice and mash until well combined.
3. Add remaining ingredients and stir to combine.
4. Divide the chicken mixture into avocado halves evenly and serve immediately.

NUTRITION: Calories: 228 Cal Fat: 13 g Carbs: 9 g Protein: 10 g Fiber: 3 g

63. Chicken & Veggie Skewers

| PREPARATION TIME: | 15' | | SERVINGS: | 6 |

| COOKING TIME: | 8' |

INGREDIENTS

- ¼ cup parmesan cheese, grated
- 3 tablespoons olive oil
- 2 garlic cloves, minced
- 1 cup fresh basil leaves, chopped
- Salt and ground black pepper, to taste
- 1¼ pounds grass-fed boneless, skinless chicken breast, cut into 1-inch cubes
- 1 large green bell pepper, seeded and cubed
- 24 cherry tomatoes

DIRECTIONS

1. Add cheese, butter, garlic, basil, salt, and black pepper in a food processor and pulse until smooth.
2. Transfer the basil mixture into a large bowl.
3. Add the chicken cubes and mix well.
4. Cover the bowl and refrigerate to marinate for at least 4–5 hours.
5. Preheat the grill to medium-high heat. Generously, grease the grill grate.
6. Strand the chicken, bell pepper cubes, and tomatoes onto presoaked woody skewers.
7. Place the skewers onto the grill and cook for about 6–8 minutes, flipping occasionally.
8. Remove from the grill and place onto a plate for about 5 minutes before serving.

NUTRITION: Calories: 201 Cal Fat: 19 g Carbs: 8 g Protein: 9 g Fiber: 4 g

64. STUFFED TOMATOES

| PREPARATION TIME: | 15' | | SERVINGS: | 10 |

| COOKING TIME: | 15' |

INGREDIENTS

- 1 pound gluten-free sausage, links removed and crumbled
- 10 medium tomatoes
- 3 tablespoons olive oil
- 10 thin Monterey Jack cheese slices
- ½ cup Monterey Jack cheese, shredded
- 2 tablespoons fresh chives, chopped finely

DIRECTIONS

1. Preheat the oven to 350°F.
2. Heat a lightly greased wok over medium heat and cook the sausage for about 6–8 minutes.
3. Eliminate from the heat and drain off any grease from sausage meat.
4. Carefully, cut a thin slice at the end of each tomato.
5. Now, cut the top part of each tomato and carefully, remove the core and seeds.
6. Coat the outer sides of tomatoes with oil lightly.
7. Arrange 1 cheese slice insides of each tomato and fill with cooked sausage.
8. Top with the shredded cheese.
9. Arrange the tomatoes onto a baking sheet.
10. Bake for approximately 5–8 minutes or until cheese is melted.
11. Remove the baking sheet from oven and set aside to cool for about 1–2 minutes before serving.
12. Garnish with chives and serve.

NUTRITION: Calories: 198 Cal Fat: 18 g Carbs: 7 g Protein: 8 g Fiber: 3 g

65. Crab Cakes

PREPARATION TIME: 15'		**SERVINGS:** 4
	COOKING TIME: 28'	

Ingredients

Crab Cakes:
- 2 tablespoons olive oil, divided
- ½ cup onion, chopped finely
- 3 tablespoons blanched almond flour
- ¼ cup organic egg whites
- 2 tablespoons mayonnaise
- 1 tablespoon dried parsley, crushed
- 1 teaspoon yellow mustard
- 1 teaspoon Worcestershire sauce
- 1 tablespoon Old Bay seasoning
- Salt and ground black pepper, to taste
- 1 pound lump crabmeat, drained

Salad:
- 5 cups fresh baby arugula
- 2 tomatoes, chopped
- 2 tablespoons olive oil
- Salt and ground black pepper, to taste

Directions

1. For crab cakes: Heat 2 teaspoons of olive oil in a wok over medium heat and sauté onion for about 8–10 minutes.
2. Remove the frying pan from heat and set aside to cool slightly.
3. Place cooked onion and remaining ingredients except for crabmeat in a mixing bowl and mix until well combined.
4. Add the crabmeat and mildly, stir to combine.
5. Make 8 equal-sized patties from the mixture.
6. Arrange the patties onto a foil-lined tray and refrigerate for about 30 minutes.
7. In a large frying pan, heat remaining oil over medium-low heat and cook patties in 2 batches for about 3–4 minutes per side or until desired doneness.
8. For salad: In a bowl, add all ingredients, and toss to coat well.
9. Divide salad onto serving plates and to each with 2 patties.
10. Serve immediately.

NUTRITION: Calories: 268 Cal Fat: 18 g Carbs: 7 g Protein: 8 g Fiber: 3 g

66. Pepperoni Pizza

Preparation Time: 15'	**Servings:** 8
Cooking Time: 20'	

Ingredients

- 2 cups mozzarella cheese
- 1 large organic egg
- 3 tablespoons cream cheese, softened
- ¾ cup almond flour
- 1 tablespoon psyllium husk
- 1 tablespoon Italian seasoning
- Salt and ground black pepper, to taste
- 1 teaspoon butter, melted

Directions

1. Preheat the oven to 400ºF
2. For the crust: In a microwave-safe bowl, place mozzarella cheese and microwave on High for about 90 seconds or until melted completely.
3. In the bowl of mozzarella, add eggs and cream cheese and mix until well combined.
4. Add the remaining ingredients and mix until well combined and a dough ball forms.
5. Coat the dough ball with melted butter and place it onto a smooth surface.
6. With your hands, press the dough ball into a circle.
7. Arrange the crust onto a baking sheet and bake for approximately 10 minutes.
8. Carefully, flip the side and bake for approximately 2–4 minutes.
9. Remove the crust from oven.
10. Spread the tomato sauce over the crust evenly.
11. Arrange the pepperoni slices over tomato sauce evenly and sprinkle with cheese.
12. Bake for approximately 3–5 minutes.
13. Remove the pizza from oven and sprinkle with oregano.
14. Cut into 6 equal-sized wedges and serve.

Nutrition: Calories: 198 Cal Fat: 13 g Carbs: 7 g Protein: 8 g Fiber: 3 g

67. Bacon with Mushrooms

Preparation Time: 15′	**Servings:** 2
Cooking Time: 16′	

Ingredients

- 4 bacon slices, cut into ½-inch pieces
- 2 cups fresh mushrooms, sliced
- 1 tablespoon garlic, chopped
- 2 fresh thyme sprigs

Directions

1. Heat a large cast-iron wok over medium heat and cook the bacon for about 5–6 minutes or until crispy.
2. Add the mushrooms and cook for about 4–5 minutes, stirring occasionally.
3. Stir in the garlic and thyme and cook for about 4–5 minutes, stirring occasionally.
4. Discard the thyme sprigs and serve hot.

Nutrition: Calories: 148 Cal Fat: 19 g Carbs: 7 g Protein: 10 g Fiber: 8 g

68. Shrimp with Zucchini Noodles

Preparation Time: 15'

Servings: 4

Cooking Time: 7'

Ingredients

- 2 tablespoons unsalted butter
- 1 large garlic clove, minced
- ¼ teaspoon red pepper flakes, crushed
- 1 pound medium shrimp, peeled and deveined
- Salt and ground black pepper, to taste
- 1/3 cup homemade chicken broth
- 2 medium zucchinis, spiralized with blade C
- ¼ cup cherry tomatoes, quartered

Directions

1. Heat the oil in a large wok over medium heat and sauté garlic and red pepper flakes for about 1 minute.
2. Add shrimp and black pepper and cook for about 1 minute per side.
3. Add broth and zucchini noodles and cook for about 2–3 minutes.
4. Stir in tomatoes and cook for about 2 minutes.
5. Serve hot.

Nutrition: Calories: 181 Cal Fat: 18 g Carbs: 7 g Protein: 8 g Fiber: 3 g

69. Spinach with Cottage Cheese

Preparation Time: 15'

Servings: 8

Cooking Time: 25'

Ingredients

- 2 (10-ounce) packages frozen spinach, thawed and drained
- 1½ cups water, divided
- ¼ cup sour cream
- 16-ounce cottage cheese, cut into ½-inch cubes
- 2 tablespoons butter
- 1 tablespoon onion, minced
- 1 tablespoon garlic, minced
- 1 tablespoon fresh ginger, minced
- 2 tablespoons tomato puree
- 2 teaspoons curry powder
- 2 teaspoons garam masala powder
- 2 teaspoons ground coriander
- 2 teaspoons ground cumin
- 2 teaspoons ground turmeric
- 2 teaspoons red pepper flakes, crushed
- Salt, to taste

Directions

1. Place spinach, ½ cup of water, and sour cream in a blender and pulse until pureed.
2. Transfer the spinach puree into a bowl and set aside.
3. In a large non-stick wok, melt butter over medium-low heat and sauté onion, garlic, ginger, tomato puree, spices, and salt for about 2–3 minutes.
4. Add the spinach puree and remaining water and stir to combine.
5. Adjust the heat to medium and cook for about 3–5 minutes.
6. Add cottage cheese cubes and stir to combine.
7. Adjust the heat to low and cook for about 10–15 minutes.
8. Serve hot.

Nutrition: Calories: 121 Cal Fat: 12 g Carbs: 9 g Protein: 4 g Fiber: 7 g

70. Green Chicken Curry

PREPARATION TIME: 15'		**SERVINGS:** 4

COOKING TIME: 30'

Ingredients

- 1 pound grass-fed skinless, boneless chicken breasts, cubed
- 1 tablespoon olive oil
- 2 tablespoons green curry paste
- 1 cup unsweetened coconut milk
- 1 cup homemade chicken broth
- 1 cup asparagus spears, trimmed and cut into pieces
- 1 cup green beans, neat and cut into pieces
- Salt and ground black pepper, to taste
- ¼ cup fresh basil leaves, chopped

Directions

1. In a wok, heat the oil over medium heat and sauté the curry paste for about 1–2 minutes.
2. Add the chicken and cook for about 8–10 minutes.
3. Add coconut milk and broth and take to a boil.
4. Adjust the heat low and cook for about 8–10 minutes.
5. Add the asparagus, green beans, salt, and black pepper, and cook for about 4–5 minutes or until desired doneness.
6. Serve hot.

NUTRITION: Calories: 150 Cal Fat: 13g Carbs: 17 g Protein: 9 g Fiber: 3 g

71. CREAMY PORK STEW

PREPARATION TIME: 15'

SERVINGS: 8

COOKING TIME: 95'

INGREDIENTS

- 3 tablespoons unsalted butter
- 2½ pounds boneless pork ribs, cut into ¾-inch cubes
- 1 large yellow onion, chopped
- 4 garlic cloves, crushed
- 1½ cups homemade chicken broth
- 2 (10-ounce) cans sugar-free diced tomatoes
- 2 teaspoons dried oregano
- 1 teaspoon ground cumin
- Salt, to taste
- 2 tablespoons fresh lime juice
- ½ cup sour cream

DIRECTIONS

1. In a large heavy-bottomed pan, dissolve the butter over medium-high heat and cook the pork, onions, and garlic for about 4–5 minutes or until browned.
2. Add the broth and with a wooden spoon, scrape up the browned bits.
3. Add the tomatoes, oregano, cumin, and salt, and stir to combine well
4. Adjust the temperature to medium-low and simmer, covered for about 1½ hours.
5. Stir in the sour cream and lime juice and remove from the heat.
6. Serve hot.

NUTRITION: Calories: 182 Cal Fat: 18 g Carbs: 9 g Protein: 18 g Fiber: 6 g

72. Salmon & Shrimp Stew

Preparation Time: 20'

Servings: 6

Cooking Time: 25'

Ingredients

- 2 tablespoons coconut oil
- ½ cup onion, chopped finely
- 2 garlic cloves, minced
- 1 Serrano pepper, chopped
- 1 teaspoon smoked paprika
- 24 cups fresh tomatoes, chopped
- 4 cups homemade chicken broth
- 1 pound salmon fillets, cubed
- 1 pound shrimp, peeled and deveined
- 2 tablespoons fresh lime juice
- Salt and ground black pepper, to taste
- 3 tablespoons fresh parsley, chopped

Directions

1. In a big soup pan, melt coconut oil over medium-high heat and sauté the onion for about 5–6 minutes.
2. Add the garlic, Serrano pepper, and paprika, and sauté for about 1 minute.
3. Add the tomatoes and broth and bring to a boil.
4. Adjust the heat to medium and simmer for about 5 minutes.
5. Add the salmon and simmer for about 3–4 minutes.
6. Stir in the shrimp and cook for about 4–5 minutes.
7. Stir in lemon juice, salt, and black pepper, and remove from heat.
8. Serve hot with the garnishing of parsley.

Nutrition: Calories: 168 Cal Fat: 12 g Carbs: 7.1 g Protein: 8.89 g Fiber: 3.2 g

73. CREAMY CHICKEN BAKE

PREPARATION TIME: 15'

SERVINGS: 6

COOKING TIME: 70'

INGREDIENTS

- 5 tablespoons unsalted butter, divided
- 2 small onions, sliced thinly
- 3 garlic cloves, minced
- 1 teaspoon dried tarragon, crushed
- 8 ounces' cream cheese, softened
- 1 cup homemade chicken broth, divided
- 2 tablespoons fresh lemon juice
- ½ cup heavy cream
- 1½ teaspoons Herbs de Provence
- Salt and ground black pepper, to taste
- 4 (6-ounce) grass-fed chicken breasts

DIRECTIONS

1. Preheat the oven to 3500F.
2. Grease a 13x9-inch baking plate with 1 tablespoon of butter.
3. In a wok, melt 2 tablespoons of butter over medium heat and sauté the onion, garlic, and tarragon for about 4–5 minutes.
4. Transfer the onion mixture onto a plate.
5. In the same wok, melt remaining 2 tablespoons of butter over low heat and cook the cream cheese, ½ cup of broth, and lemon juice for about 3–4 minutes, stirring continuously.
6. 6 Stir in the cream, herbs de Provence, salt, and black pepper, and remove from heat.
7. Pour remaining broth in prepared baking dish.
8. Arrange chicken breasts in the baking dish in a single layer and top with the cream mixture evenly.
9. Bake for approximately 45–60 minutes.
10. Serve hot.

NUTRITION: Calories: 129 Cal Fat: 12 g Carbs: 9 g Protein: 7 g Fiber: 5 g

74. Beef & Veggie Casserole

Preparation Time: 20'		**Servings:** 6
	Cooking Time: 55'	

Ingredients

- 3 tablespoons butter
- 1 pound grass-fed ground beef
- 1 medium yellow onion, chopped
- 2 garlic cloves, chopped
- 1 cup pumpkin, peeled and chopped
- 1 cup broccoli, chopped
- 2 cups cheddar cheese, shredded
- 1 tablespoon Dijon mustard
- 6 large organic eggs
- ½ cup heavy whipping cream
- Salt and ground black pepper, to taste

Directions

1. In a non-stick wok, melt 1 tablespoon of butter over medium heat and cook the beef for about 8–10 minutes or until no longer pink, breaking up the lumps.
2. With a positioned spoon, transfer the beef into a large bowl.
3. In the same wok, melt the remaining butter over medium heat and cook the onion and garlic for about 10 minutes, stirring frequently.
4. Add the pumpkin and cook for about 5–6 minutes.
5. Add the broccoli and cook for about 3–4 minutes.
6. Transfer the pumpkin mixture into the bowl with cooked beef and stir to combine.
7. Set aside to cool slightly.
8. Meanwhile, preheat the oven to 350°F.
9. In the bowl of beef mixture, add 2/3 of cheese and mustard and stir to combine.
10. In another mixing bowl, add cream, eggs, salt, and black pepper, and beat until well combined.
11. In a baking dish, place the beef mixture and top with egg mixture, followed by the remaining cheese.
12. Bake for approximately 25 minutes or until the top becomes golden brown.
13. Remove the baking dish from oven and set aside for about 5 minutes before serving.
14. Cut into desired-sized wedges and serve.

Nutrition: Calories: 210 Cal Fat: 18 g Carbs: 7 g Protein: 8 g Fiber: 3 g

75. Beef with Bell Peppers

Preparation Time: 15'

Cooking Time: 10'

Servings: 4

Ingredients

- 1 tablespoon olive oil
- 1 pound grass-fed flank steak, cut into thin slices across the grain diagonally
- 1 red bell pepper, seeded and cut into thin strips
- 1 green bell pepper, seeded and cut into thin strips
- 1 tablespoon fresh ginger, minced
- 3 tablespoons low-sodium soy sauce
- 1½ tablespoons balsamic vinegar
- 2 teaspoons Sriracha

Directions

1. In a big non-stick wok, heat the oil over medium-high heat and sear the steak slices for about 2 minutes.
2. Add bell peppers and cook for about 2–3 minutes, stirring continuously.
3. With a slotted spoon, transfer the beef mixture into a bowl.
4. the wok, add the remaining ingredients over medium heat, and bring to a boil.
5. Cook for about 1 minute, stirring frequently.
6. Add the beef mixture and cook for about 1–2 minutes.
7. Serve hot.

Nutrition: Calories: 271 Cal Fat: 10 g Carbs: 8 g Protein: 19 g Fiber: 3 g

76. Coconut Keto Porridge

PREPARATION TIME:	5'		SERVINGS:	2

COOKING TIME: 10'

INGREDIENTS

- 4 tbsp. of coconut cream
- 1 pinch of ground psyllium husk powder
- 1 tbsp. of coconut flour
- 1 flaxseed egg
- 1 oz. of coconut butter

DIRECTIONS

1. Toss all of the fixings together in a small pan before placing the pan on the stovetop burner set to low heat.
2. Stir the mixture as it cooks to encourage the porridge to thicken. Continue stirring until your preferred thickness is reached.
3. A small amount of coconut milk or a few berries (fresh or frozen) can also be added to taste if desired.

NUTRITION: Calories: 408 Cal Fat: 20 g Carbs: 4 g Protein: 8 g Fiber: 3 g

77. Cream Cheese Eggs

Preparation Time: 5'

Servings: 2

Cooking Time: 5'

Ingredients

- 1 tbsp. of butter
- 2 eggs
- 2 tbsp. of soft cream cheese with chives

Directions

1. Preheat a skillet and melt the butter.
2. Whisk the eggs with the cream cheese.
3. Add to the pan and stir until done.

Nutrition: Calories: 308 Cal Fat: 12 g Carbs: 4 g Protein: 9 g Fiber: 5 g

78. Creamy Basil Baked Sausage

Preparation Time:	5'	
		Servings: 2
	Cooking Time: 30'	

Ingredients

- 3 lb. of Italian sausage - pork/turkey or chicken
- 8 ozs. of cream cheese
- .25 cup of heavy cream
- .25 cup of basil pesto
- 8 g of mozzarella

Directions

1. Set the oven at 400° Fahrenheit.
2. Lightly spritz a casserole dish with cooking oil spray. Add the sausage to the dish and bake for 30 minutes.
3. Combine the heavy cream, pesto, and cream cheese.
4. Pour the sauce over the casserole and top it off with the cheese.
5. Bake for another 10 minutes. The sausage should reach 160° Fahrenheit in the center when checked with a meat thermometer.
6. You can also broil for 3 minutes to brown the cheesy layer.

Nutrition: Calories: 298 Cal Fat: 17 g Carbs: 4 g Protein: 9 g Fiber: 3 g

79. KETO BRUNCH SPREAD

PREPARATION TIME: 5′

SERVINGS: 4

COOKING TIME: 20′

INGREDIENTS

- 4 large eggs
- 24 asparagus spears
- 12 slices of sugar-free bacon

DIRECTIONS

1. Set the oven at 400° Fahrenheit.
2. Slender the asparagus about one inch from the bottoms.
3. In pairs, wrap them with one slice of bacon.
4. Firmly hold the spears in one hand as you wind the bacon slices from the bottom to the top. Pull the bacon tightly and arrange on a baking tin.
5. Repeat until you have 12 pairs.
6. Set the oven timer for 20 minutes.
7. Now, start a pot of water to a rapid boil. Place the eggs gently in the boiling water. Boil for six minutes.
8. Fill a bowl with ice water and add the eggs for another two minutes before removing the peeling from the tops/tips.
9. When the asparagus is ready, serve on a cutting board/tray. You can use an espresso cup if you don't have an egg holder to keep the eggs sitting upright.
10. Use a small spoon to scoop out the tops of the soft-boiled eggs to reveal the runny yolk.
11. Dip the asparagus into the yolks. Enjoy the egg white with some keto-friendly toast.

NUTRITION: Calories: 309 Cal Fat: 10 g Carbs: 4 g Protein: 8 g Fiber: 3 g

80. Mushroom Omelet

Preparation Time: 5'

Servings: 3

Cooking Time: 10'

Ingredients

- 1 oz. of butter
- 3 eggs
- 1 oz. of shredded cheese
- 3 tbsp. of yellow onion
- 3 mushrooms

Directions

1. Whisk the eggs, salt, and pepper until frothy. Sprinkle in the spices.
2. Add the butter to a skillet. When melted, add the eggs.
3. Prepare the omelet. Once the bottom is firm, sprinkle with onions, mushrooms, and cheese.
4. Carefully remove the edges and fold the omelet in half.
5. Slide onto the plate when done to serve.

Nutrition: Calories: 309 Cal Fat: 10 g Carbs: 2 g Protein: 9 g Fiber: 4 g

81. 1-Minute Keto Muffins

PREPARATION TIME: 5'

SERVINGS: 3

COOKING TIME: 35'

INGREDIENTS

- 1 egg
- A pinch of salt
- 2 tbsp. of coconut flour
- 1 pinch of baking soda
- Butter/coconut oil (as needed)

DIRECTIONS

1. Lightly grease a large coffee mug/ramekin dish using butter or coconut
2. oil/butter.
3. Whisk all of the fixings together and cook for one minute using high for 45 seconds to one minute in the microwave. You can also bake for 12 minutes at 400° Fahrenheit in the oven.
4. Slice in half or toast and serve.

NUTRITION: Calories: 172 Cal Fat: 4 g Carbs: 2 g Protein: 5 g Fiber: 2 g

82. PEANUT BUTTER PROTEIN BARS

PREPARATION TIME: 5'	SERVINGS: 12

COOKING TIME: 15'

INGREDIENTS

- 1.5 cups of almond meal
- 1 cup of Keto-friendly chunky peanut butter
- 2 egg whites
- .5 cup of almonds
- .5 cup of cashews
- Also needed: baking pan

DIRECTIONS

1. Heat the oven ahead of time to reach 350° Fahrenheit.
2. Spritz a baking dish lightly with coconut or olive oil.
3. Combine all of the fixings and add them to the prepared dish.
4. Bake for 15 minutes and then cut into 12 pieces once they're cool.
5. Store in the refrigerator to keep them fresh.

NUTRITION: Calories: 506 Cal Fat: 18g Carbs: 5 g Protein: 19 g Fiber: 2 g

83. Tuna Stuffed Avocado

Preparation Time: 10′	**Servings:** 4

Cooking Time: 0′

Ingredients

- 2 tbsp. of Greek yogurt/mayonnaise
- 5 ozs. can drained tuna
- Medium avocado
- 1 pinch of dried dill

Directions

1. Combine the fixings (mayo, tuna, and dill).
2. Cut the avocado in half and eliminate the pit. Fill it with the salad and serve.

Nutrition: Calories: 401 Cal Fat: 20 g Carbs: 4 g Protein: 8 g Fiber: 3 g

84. Bacon Burger Cabbage Stir Fry

Preparation Time: 5′	**Servings:** 10
Cooking Time: 20′	

Ingredients

- 1 lb. of ground beef
- 1 lb. of bacon
- 1 small onion
- 3 minced cloves of garlic
- 1 lb./1 small head of cabbage

Directions

1. Dice the bacon and onion.
2. Combine the beef and bacon in a wok or large skillet. Prepare it until done and store it in a bowl to keep warm.
3. Mince the onion and garlic. Toss both into the hot grease.
4. Slice and toss in the cabbage and stir-fry until wilted.
5. Blend in the meat and combine. Sprinkle with pepper and salt as desired.

Nutrition: Calories: 357 Cal Fat: 22 g Carbs: 6 g Protein: 20 g Fiber: 4 g

85. Bacon Cheeseburger

Preparation Time: 5'

Servings: 12

Cooking Time: 0'

Ingredients

- 16 ozs. pkg. of low-sodium bacon
- 3 lbs. of ground beef
- 2 eggs
- Half of 1 medium chopped onion
- 8 ozs. of shredded cheddar cheese

Directions

1. Fry the bacon and chop it to bits. Shred the cheese and dice the onion.
2. Combine the mixture with the beef and blend in the whisked eggs.
3. Prepare 24 burgers and grill them the way you like them.
4. You can make a double-decker since they are small. If you like a bigger burger, you can make 12 burgers as a single-decker.

Nutrition: Calories: 489 Cal Fat: 21 g Carbs: 4 g Protein: 26 g Fiber: 3 g

86. Cauliflower Mac & Cheese

Preparation Time: 10'

Servings: 4

Cooking Time: 15'

Ingredients

- 1 head of cauliflower
- 3 tbsp. of butter
- .25 cup of unsweetened almond milk
- .25 cup of heavy cream
- 1 cup of cheddar cheese

Directions

1. Use a sharp knife to slice the cauliflower into small florets. Shred the cheese.
2. Prepare the oven to reach 450° Fahrenheit.
3. Cover a baking pan with a layer of parchment baking paper or foil.
4. Add two tablespoons of the butter to a pan and melt. Add the florets, butter, salt, and pepper together. Place the cauliflower on the baking pan and roast 10 to 15 minutes.
5. Warm up the rest of the butter, milk, heavy cream, and cheese in the microwave or double boiler. Pour the cheese over the cauliflower and serve.

Nutrition: Calories: 298 Cal Fat: 20 g Carbs: 4 g Protein: 8 g Fiber: 3 g

87. Mushroom & Cauliflower Risotto

Preparation Time: 15′

Servings: 2

Cooking Time: 10′

Ingredients

- 1 grated head of cauliflower
- 1 cup of vegetable stock
- 9 ozs. of chopped mushrooms
- 2 tbsp. of butter
- 1 cup of coconut cream

Directions

1. Pour the stock in a saucepan. Boil and set aside.
2. Prepare a skillet with butter and saute the mushrooms until golden.
3. Grate and stir in the cauliflower and stock.
4. Simmer and add the cream, cooking until the cauliflower is al dente. Serve.

Nutrition: Calories: 186 Cal Fat: 12 g Carbs: 4 g Protein: 9 g Fiber: 3 g

88. Skillet Cabbage Tacos

Preparation Time: 5'	**Servings:** 4

Cooking Time: 12'

Ingredients

- 1 lb. of ground beef
- .5 cup of salsa - ex. Pace Organic
- 2 cups of shredded cabbage
- 2 tbsp. of chili powder
- .75 cup of shredded cheese

Directions

1. Brown the beef and drain the fat. Pour in the salsa, cabbage, and seasoning.
2. Cover and lower the heat. Simmer for 10 to 12 minutes using the medium heat temperature setting.
3. When the cabbage has softened, remove it from the heat and mix in the cheese.
4. Top it off using your favorite toppings, such as green onions or sour cream, and serve.

Nutrition: Calories: 328 Cal Fat: 21 g Carbs: 4 g Protein: 18 g Fiber: 3 g

89. Chicken-Pecan Salad & Cucumber Bites

Preparation Time: 5'

Servings: 4

Cooking Time: 0'

Ingredients

- 1 cucumber
- 1 cup of precooked chicken breast
- .25 cup of celery
- 2 tbsp. of mayonnaise
- .25 cup of pecans

Directions

1. Peel and slice the cucumber into .25-inch slices. Dice the chicken and celery. Chop the pecans. Combine the pecans, chicken, mayonnaise, and celery in a salad bowl. Sprinkle with pepper and salt if desired.
2. Prepare the cucumber slices. Layer each one with a spoonful of the chicken salad. Serve.

Nutrition: Calories: 323 Cal Fat: 24 g Carbs: 5 g Protein: 4 g Fiber: 6 g

90. Curry Egg Salad

Preparation Time: 5'

Servings: 6

Cooking Time: 0'

Ingredients

- 6 hard-boiled eggs
- 1 tbsp. or to taste of curry powder
- .5 cup of full-fat mayonnaise

Directions

1. Prepare the boiled eggs by adding them into a saucepan. Pour in cold water. Turn the burner on.
2. Wait for the water to boil and set a timer for seven minutes.
3. Empty the hot water and place the eggs in a dish of cold water/ice to hinder the cooking process.
4. Once they're cool, peel and chop the eggs into small bits.
5. Combine the mayo, eggs, and curry powder.
6. Serve with a portion of chopped fresh parsley.

Nutrition: Calories: 80 Cal Fat: 5 g Carbs: 4 g Protein: 8 g Fiber: 3 g

91. Keto-Cauli Tots

| PREPARATION TIME: | 20' | | SERVINGS: | 4 |

| COOKING TIME: | 18' |

INGREDIENTS

- 2 cups cauliflower, steamed and destroyed
- 8 tbsp. destroyed parmesan cheddar
- 1 tbsp. spread
- 1 huge egg
- 1/4 tsp onion powder
- Salt and pepper, to taste

DIRECTIONS

1. Preheat your stove to 425 °F.
2. Consolidate all fixings in an enormous bowl and blend well.
3. With a teaspoon scoop a potato size spoon full and shape into the ideal potato.
4. Refrigerate tots for 10 minutes or until firm.
5. Prepare for approx. 18 minutes, or until brilliant and fresh. Appreciate!

NUTRITION: Calories: 170 Cal Fat: 22 g Carbs: 7 g Protein: 9 g Fiber: 3 g

92. Spicy Sausage and Portobello Pizza's Plans

Preparation Time: 5'	**Servings:** 6
Cooking Time: 15'	

Ingredients

- 6 portobellos, stemmed
- Salt and pepper
- 2 tablespoons olive oil
- 1 medium onion, slashed
- 1 clove garlic, minced
- 12 ounces hot Italian frankfurter, packaging expelled
- 3 medium tomatoes, stripped, seeded and diced
- 1 teaspoon slashed new oregano (or 1/2 tsp. dried)
- 1/4 teaspoon squashed red pepper
- 3/4 cup destroyed mozzarella

Directions

1. Preheat broiler to 375°F. Holding a portobello in 1 hand, utilize a little spoon to tenderly scratch out gills from the underside.
2. Rehash with rest of mushrooms.
3. Sprinkle with salt and pepper.
4. Spot portobellos level, gill side down, on an enormous preparing sheet; heat until somewhat mellowed and simply starting to radiate fluid, 10 to 15 minutes. (Time will shift as indicated by size of portobellos.)
5. Pat gill side dry with paper towels.
6. Warm oil in an enormous skillet over medium-high warmth.
7. Cook onion, blending, until mollified, 3 to 5 minutes.
8. Include garlic; sauté brief more.
9. Include frankfurter and cook, separating enormous pieces, until never again pink, 5 to 7 minutes.
10. Mix in tomatoes and increment warmth to high. Cook, mixing, until fluid has vanished, 10 to 12 minutes.
11. Mix in oregano and red pepper. Season with salt and pepper.
12. Gap frankfurter blend among portobellos, filling gill side of each with around 1/2 cup. Top with mozzarella.
13. Prepare until cooked through and cheddar is dissolved, around 10 minutes. Serve right away.

Nutrition: Calories: 298 Cal Fat: 20 g Carbs: 4 g Protein: 8 g Fiber: 3 g

93. Chicken and Prosciutto Salad with Arugula and Asiago

Preparation Time: 15'

Servings: 6

Cooking Time: 20'

Ingredients

- 2 (1-ounce) cuts sourdough bread, cut into 1/2-inch solid shapes cooking splash
- 1/2 teaspoon dried basil
- 1/8 teaspoon garlic powder
- 3 tablespoons extra-virgin olive oil, partitioned
- 2 ounces' slender cuts prosciutto, cleaved
- 2 tablespoons crisp lemon juice
- 1/4 teaspoon salt
- 2 (5-ounce) bundles infant arugula
- 1/2 ounces Asiago cheddar, shaved and separated (around 1/3 cup)
- 6 ounces destroyed skinless, boneless rotisserie chicken bosom
- 1 cup grape tomatoes, split.

Directions

1. Preheat broiler to 425°.
2. Spot bread shapes on a preparing sheet, and gently cover with cooking shower.
3. Include basil and garlic powder; hurl well. Spot bread blend in preheating broiler; heat for 8 minutes or until fresh.
4. Medium-high warmth.
5. Add 1 teaspoon oil to the dish; whirl to cover. Include prosciutto; sauté 4 minutes or until prosciutto is fresh. Channel on paper towels.
6. Consolidate staying 2 tablespoons in addition to 2 teaspoons oil, squeeze, and salt in a little bowl; mix well with a whisk. Spot arugula, half of cheddar, and juice blend in an enormous bowl; hurl well to cover.
7. Partition arugula blends equally among 6 plates; isolate chicken, prosciutto, tomatoes, remaining cheddar, and bread garnishes equitably over servings of mixed greens.

Nutrition: Calories: 128 Cal Fat: 13 g Carbs: 4 g Protein: 7 g Fiber: 2 g

94. Caesar Brussels Grows with Almonds Salad.

Preparation Time: 11'

Servings: 4

Cooking Time: 12'

Ingredients

- 2 tablespoons cut almonds
- 2 tablespoons new lemon juice
- 1/2 teaspoon dark pepper dash of legitimate salt
- 2 garlic cloves, finely cleaved
- 1/2 tablespoons olive oil
- 2 tablespoons finely ground Parmesan cheddar
- 1 (12-ozs.) pkg. shaved new Brussels grows

Directions

1. Warmth a huge nonstick skillet over medium-high.
2. Include cut almonds, and cook 4 minutes or until toasted and fragrant, mixing once in a while.
3. Consolidate lemon juice, pepper, fit salt, and cleaved garlic in a bowl; let stand 5 minutes.
4. Include olive oil and Parmesan cheddar to bowl, mixing with a whisk. Include almonds and Brussels grows; hurl to cover.
5. Serve right away.

Nutrition: Calories: 238 Cal Fat: 26 g Carbs: 6 g Protein: 7 g Fiber: 3 g

95. Chicken Pan-Grilled with Chorizo Confetti

| PREPARATION TIME: | 5' | | SERVINGS: | 4 |

| COOKING TIME: | 30' |

INGREDIENTS

- 4 (6-ounce) skinless, boneless chicken bosom parts
- 1/2 teaspoon genuine salt, isolated
- 1/4 teaspoon newly ground dark pepper Cooking splash
- 1/4 cup Mexican pork chorizo, housings expelled
- 1/4 cup cut onion 2 tablespoons diced carrot
- 1/4 cup diced yellow ringer pepper
- 1/4 cup diced red chime pepper
- 2 tablespoons diced green chime pepper
- 1/4 cup unsalted chicken stock
- 1 tablespoon cleaved new cilantro Green Salad with Simple Vinaigrette Goat Cheese & Crostini.

DIRECTIONS

1. Warmth a flame broil skillet over medium-high warmth.
2. Sprinkle chicken with 1/4 teaspoon salt and pepper.
3. Coat dish with cooking splash.
4. Add chicken to the dish; cook 6 minutes on each side or until done.
5. While chicken cooks, heat a huge skillet over medium-high warmth. Include chorizo; cook 1 moment, mixing to disintegrate.
6. Include staying 1/4 teaspoon salt, onion, and carrot; cook 2 minutes, blending infrequently.
7. Include chime peppers; cook 1 moment or until fresh delicate. Include stock; cook 2 minutes or until fluid nearly vanishes, scratching container to slacken sautéed bits.
8. Spoon chorizo blend over chicken; top with cilantro.

NUTRITION: Calories: 190 Cal Fat: 22 g Carbs: 5 g Protein: 12 g Fiber: 3 g

96. Salmon with Pesto, Red Pepper

Preparation Time: 10'

Servings: 4

Cooking Time: 25'

Ingredients

- 2 chime peppers, daintily cut
- 1 little red onion, meagerly cut
- 4 cuts bread, torn
- 2 tablespoons olive oil
- 4 6-ounce skinless salmon filets legitimate
- salt and dark pepper
- 1/4 cup pesto.

Directions

1. Warmth stove to 450° F.
2. On a rimmed preparing sheet, hurl the peppers, onion, and bread with the oil.
3. Settle salmon filets in the blend; season with ¾ teaspoon salt and ¼ teaspoon pepper.
4. Broil until the salmon is misty all through and the vegetables are delicate, 8 to 10 minutes.
5. Serve bested with the pesto.

Nutrition: Calories: 318 Cal Fat: 22 g Carbs: 5 g Protein: 7 g Fiber: 4 g

97. LEMONY SHRIMP GRILLED PLATE OF MIXED GREENS

PREPARATION TIME: 5'

SERVINGS: 4

COOKING TIME: 30'

INGREDIENTS

- 1/2 lemon, in addition to
- 2 tablespoons crisp lemon juice
- 1/2 teaspoon dark peppercorns Salt
- 1 pound shelled and deveined medium shrimp
- 2 tablespoons extra-virgin olive oil
- 2 tablespoons grapeseed or vegetable oil pinch of sugar freshly ground pepper
- 2 hearts of romaine, cut into 1-inch-wide strips
- 1 cup grape tomatoes, split
- 1 Hass avocado, diced
- 2 tablespoons cut chives

DIRECTIONS

1. Fill a medium pot with water.
2. Crush the lemon half into the water, at that point add it to the water with the peppercorns and a liberal spot of salt; heat to the point of boiling.
3. Include the shrimp and stew until twisted and simply pink, around 3 minutes.
4. Utilizing an opened spoon, move the shrimp to a paper towel-lined plate.
5. Freeze the shrimp until just chilled, around 5 minutes.
6. In the interim, in an enormous bowl, whisk the lemon juice with the olive oil, grapeseed oil, sugar and a liberal squeeze every one of salt and pepper. Include the romaine, tomatoes, avocado and shrimp and hurl. Move to plates, decorate with the chives and serve.

NUTRITION: Calories: 189 Cal Fat: 19 g Carbs: 4 g Protein: 9 g Fiber: 4 g

98. Roasted Red Pepper and Chicken

Preparation Time: 5'	**Servings:** 2

Cooking Time: 40'

Ingredients

- 1 tsp. prepared salt blend
- 1 oz. balsamic vinegar
- 8 ozs. brussels sprouts
- 13 ozs. boneless skinless chicken breasts
- 1 red onion
- 2 ozs. broiled red peppers
- 4 ozs. light cream
- 1 tsp. sugar

Directions

1. Set up the Ingredients: Trim stems off Brussels sprouts and cut into flimsy strips. Divide and strip onion. Cut parts into meager strips. Mince broiled red peppers. Pat chicken bosoms dry, and season the two sides with prepared salt.
2. Start the Brussels Sprouts: Spot Brussels grows on the arranged heating sheet and hurl with 2 tsp. olive oil and ¼ tsp. salt. Spread into a solitary layer on one side and dish in a hot stove, 5 minutes. Expel from the stove. Brussels sprouts will complete the process of cooking in a later advance. While Brussels grows cook, singe chicken.
3. Cook Chicken and Finish Brussels Sprouts: Spot a medium non-stick skillet over medium warmth and include 1 tsp. olive oil. Add chicken bosoms to hot skillet and cook undisturbed until caramelized, 4-5 minutes. Move chicken, singed side up, to purge half of heating the sheet. Broil until chicken arrives at the very least interior temperature of 165 degrees, 8-10 minutes. Wipe skillet clean and hold. While chicken dishes, make onion jam.
4. Make the Onion Jam: Spot an enormous non-stick dish over medium-high warmth and include 2 tsp. olive oil. Add onion to hot container and mix once in a while until caramelized, 6-8 minutes. Mix in sugar and balsamic vinegar and cook until fluid is nearly dissipated 30-60 seconds. Expel from the burner.
5. Make Sauce and Finish Dish: Return dish used to cook the chicken to medium warmth and include 1 tsp. olive oil. Add broiled red peppers to hot dish and cook until warm, 30-60 seconds. Include cream and a touch of salt and heat to the point of boiling. When bubbling, mix at times until thickened, 2-3 minutes

Nutrition: Calories: 310 Cal Fat: 28 g Carbs: 7 g Protein: 21 g Fiber: 3 g

99. Sausage Patties with Spinach

PREPARATION TIME: 5'		**SERVINGS:** 4

COOKING TIME: 30'

Ingredients

- 10 ounces' infant spinach
- 2 tablespoons extra-virgin olive oil, in addition to additional for brushing
- 2 garlic cloves, minced
- 1 teaspoon anchovy glue (discretionary)
- Salt
- 1 pound sweet or blistering Italian hotdogs (or a blend of both), housings evacuated
- 4 cuts of provolone cheddar
- 1/4 cup sun-dried tomato pesto
- 4 round crusty bread moves, split and toasted
- 4 round crusty bread moves, split and toasted

Directions

1. In a huge skillet, bring 1/4 inch of water to a bubble. Include the spinach and cook, mixing, until simply withered, around 1 moment; channel and press out however much water as could reasonably be expected. Crash the skillet.
2. In a similar skillet, heat the 2 tablespoons of olive oil until sparkling. Include the garlic and anchovy glue and cook over high warmth, blending, until fragrant, 1 moment. Include the spinach, season with salt and mix just until covered, around 10 seconds.
3. Light a barbecue or preheat a flame broil skillet. Utilizing somewhat soaked hands, structure the hotdog meat into four 4-inch patties, around 3/4 inch thick. Brush the burgers with oil and flame broil over moderate warmth until cooked and dried up on the base, around 5 minutes. Cautiously flip the burgers. Top with the cheddar and flame broil until the burgers are cooked through and the cheddar is softened, around 5 minutes longer. Spread the pesto on the rolls. Top with the burgers and spinach and serve.

NUTRITION: Calories: 298 Cal Fat: 20 g Carbs: 4 g Protein: 8 g Fiber: 3 g

100. Broiled Salmon and Asparagus with Crème Fraiche

Preparation Time: 5'

Servings: 4

Cooking Time: 30'

Ingredients

- 2 bundles asparagus (around 2 lbs. absolute)
- 3 tablespoons extra-virgin olive oil About
- 3/4 tsp. legitimate salt, separated About
- 1/2 tsp. pepper, isolated
- 4 cleaned salmon filets (5 to 6 ozs. every)
- 1/2 cup Crème Fraîche
- 1 tablespoon every entire grain mustard and hacked crisp chives

Directions

1. Preheat grill with broiler rack around 4 in. from heat.
2. Snap off the base of an asparagus lance to see where it breaks no problem at all. Line up outstanding lances and cut off bottoms at a similar spot. Put cut asparagus on a 12-by 17-in. rimmed preparing sheet, sprinkle with oil and 1/4 tsp. each salt and pepper, and hurl to cover. Organize asparagus in a solitary layer on preparing sheet.
3. Season salmon with staying 1/2 tsp. salt and 1/4 tsp. pepper, at that point set on asparagus in a solitary layer.
4. Sear salmon and asparagus until salmon is never again translucent yet at the same time wet in focus and asparagus is sautéed in spots, 8 to 12 minutes. In the event that asparagus isn't done, lift salmon to a platter and return asparagus to broiler for a couple of more minutes.
5. Then, whisk together Crème Fraîche, mustard, chives, and salt and pepper to taste in a little bowl.
6. Serve salmon and asparagus with Crème Fraîche sauce.

Nutrition: Calories: 298 Cal Fat: 20 g Carbs: 4 g Protein: 8 g Fiber: 3 g

101. FLANK STEAK SKILLET BARBECUED

PREPARATION TIME: 15'

SERVINGS: 4-6

COOKING TIME: 10'

INGREDIENTS

- Crude flank steak on butcher paper
- 1/2 pound flank steak
- Salt
- Naturally ground dark pepper
- Dry mustard
- Relaxed margarine

DIRECTIONS

1. Tenderize the steak with shallow cuts: Remove the steak from the fridge a half hour before cooking.
2. Remove any extreme connective tissue on the outside of the steak.
3. Utilizing the tip of a sharp blade, stick little cuts into the meat, practically completely through. The cuts ought to be at an edge, toward the grain of the meat as the blade tip is going in. The cuts ought to be about an inch separated from one another.
4. Turn the steak over and rehash the cuts on the opposite side. Ensure that the cuts you are making on this side are corresponding with the cuts you made on the opposite side, else you may cut over a current cut, and wind up jabbing a gap through the meat.
5. Rub with salt, pepper, dry mustard, and spread: Sprinkle one side of the steak with salt and crisply ground pepper. Sprinkle the steak with dry mustard. Rub a tablespoon of margarine everywhere throughout the side of the steak. Turn the steak over and rehash with the dry mustard, pepper, and margarine. Rub flank steak with dry mustard rub flank steak with spread
6. Sear steak in hot skillet: Heat an enormous cast iron griddle on high warmth. Spot steak in hot container. Let singe for 2 to 3 minutes until very much cooked.
7. Place flank steak in fricasseeing pan sear flank steak in griddle
8. Go through tongs to lift to check whether pleasantly caramelized. Assuming this is the case, flip to the opposite side and let burn for 2 to 3 minutes.
9. Turn flank steak over in pan sear flank steak in skillet

10. Remove from heat: Remove the skillet from the warmth and let the steak keep on cooking for 5 to 10 minutes in the lingering warmth of the container (expecting you are utilizing solid metal, if not, bring down the warmth to low).
11. Check for doneness: Use your fingertips to check for doneness or embed a meat thermometer into the thickest piece of the steak - 120°F for uncommon, 125°F for uncommon, or 130°F for medium uncommon. Flank steak ought to be served uncommon or medium uncommon, else it might be excessively dry.
12. In the event that the steak isn't done what's necessary just as you would prefer, return the steak and container to medium high warmth for a couple of moments.
13. Let the steak rest: Remove the steak from the dish to a cutting board and let rest for 10 minutes, secured with aluminum foil.
14. Thinly cut: Cut the meat in slim cuts, at an edge, over the grain of the meat. (Along these lines you get through the extreme long muscle strands.)
15. Cutting flank steak: 8 Boil juices, deglaze skillet, add margarine to make sauce: Any juices that leave the meat while cutting or resting, come back to the dish. Return the skillet to a burner on high warmth and deglaze the container with a little water, scraping up any sautéed bits. When the water has generally come down, add a little margarine to the prospect pleasant sauce.
16. Orchestrate the cut meat on a serving plate and pour the deglazed container squeezes over the meat.

NUTRITION: Calories: 128 Cal Fat: 21 g Carbs: 4 g Protein: 2 g Fiber: 5 g

102. Avocados stuffed with Crap

PREPARATION TIME:	20'		SERVINGS:	4

COOKING TIME: 50'

INGREDIENTS

- 1 pound boneless, skinless chicken bosom
- 1/3 cup low-fat plain Greek yogurt
- ¼ cup mayonnaise
- 1 tablespoon slashed crisp tarragon or 1 teaspoon dried
- ¾ teaspoon salt
- ½ teaspoon ground pepper
- 1 cup diced celery
- 1 cup seedless red grapes, divided (discretionary)
- ¼ cup toasted slashed walnuts
- 2 firm ready avocados, divided and pitted

DIRECTIONS

1. Spot chicken in an enormous pan and add enough water to cover. Bring to a stew over medium warmth. Diminish warmth to keep up a stew, spread and cook until the chicken registers 165 degrees F with a moment read thermometer, 12 to 15 minutes. Move to a cutting board. Let remain until sufficiently cool to deal with, at that point hack or shred. Refrigerate until chilly, around 30 minutes.
2. To serve, fill every avocado half with around 1/2 cup chicken plate of mixed greens. (Refrigerate the additional chicken plate of mixed greens for as long as 3 days.)

NUTRITION: Calories: 308 Cal Fat: 22 g Carbs: 6 g Protein: 8 g Fiber: 4 g

103. BLACKENED CHICKEN SALAD

| PREPARATION TIME: | 5' | | SERVINGS: | 4 |

| COOKING TIME: | 0' |

INGREDIENTS

- 2 cups cooked chicken bosom, slashed
- 4 tbsp. nonfat plain yogurt (or low-fat mayonnaise)
- 4 tbsp. low fat harsh cream
- 2 tsps. nectar
- 1 cup destroyed carrots
- 1/2 cup green onions, minced
- 1 tbsp. lemon juice
- 1 tsp. paprika
- 1/2 tsp. garlic powder
- 1/2 tsp. onion powder
- 1/2 tsp. dark pepper
- 1/2 tsp. oregano
- 1/2 tsp. cumin
- 1/8 tsp. cayenne pepper (or more)
- Salt to taste

DIRECTIONS

1. Combine the yogurt, harsh cream, lemon, nectar, and all the flavors.
2. Include the chicken, carrots, and green onions.
3. Taste and season with salt, pepper, or cayenne.

NUTRITION: Calories: 173 Cal Fat: 21 g Carbs: 5 g Protein: 6 gFiber: 2 g

104. Vinaigrette with Blue Cheese

PREPARATION TIME:	5'		SERVINGS:	2

COOKING TIME: 5'

Ingredients

- 2 hearts romaine, hacked
- 1 clove garlic, hacked
- 1/2 teaspoon dried oregano leaves
- 2 teaspoons sugar
- 2 tablespoons red wine vinegar
- 1/4 cup extra-virgin olive oil
- 1/4 pound blue cheddar disintegrates, in claim to fame cheddar segment of your market
- Salt and pepper

Directions

1. Spot lettuce in a major bowl. Consolidate garlic, oregano, sugar and vinegar in a little bowl.
2. Add oil to dressing in a moderate stream and blend in with a whisk or fork and mix in blue cheddar.
3. Pour dressing over plate of mixed greens and hurl.
4. Season with salt and pepper, to taste.

NUTRITION: Calories: 128 Cal Fat: 16 g Carbs: 2 g Protein: 5 g Fiber: 2.1 g

105. Mint Raita grilled Chicken with Tandoori

Preparation Time: 20'

Servings: 4

Cooking Time: 45'

Ingredients

- 2 tablespoons hacked stripped new ginger
- 1 tablespoon paprika
- 1 tablespoon new lime juice
- 1 teaspoon stew powder
- 3/4 teaspoon salt
- 1/2 teaspoon ground turmeric
- 1/2 teaspoon ground cumin
- 1/8 teaspoon ground red pepper
- 3 garlic cloves, cleaved
- 4 (12-ounce) bone-in chicken leg-thigh quarters, cleaned Raita:
- 3/4 cup sans fat Greek yogurt
- 3/4 cup slashed seeded cucumber
- 2 tablespoons cleaved crisp mint
- 1/2 teaspoon ground cumin
- 1/4 teaspoon salt Cooking shower

Directions

1. To set up the marinade, join initial 10 fixings in a blender; process until smooth. Fill an enormous zip-top plastic sack. Include chicken; go to cover. Marinate chicken in cooler for at any rate 4 hours or medium-term.
2. To set up the raita, join 3/4 cup yogurt and remaining fixings aside from cooking shower in a little bowl; cover and refrigerate.
3. Expel chicken from the cooler, and let remain at room temperature for 45 minutes.
4. Set up the flame broil for aberrant barbecuing. On the off chance that utilizing a gas flame broil, heat one side to medium-high and leave one side with no warmth. On the off chance that utilizing a charcoal barbecue, orchestrate hot coals on either side of the charcoal mesh, leaving an unfilled space in the center.
5. Expel the chicken from marinade, and dispose of the rest of the marinade. Spot the chicken on an unheated piece of flame broil rack covered with cooking shower. Close top, and barbecue for an hour and a half or until a thermometer embedded into a substantial piece of the thigh register 165°, turning chicken like clockwork.

NUTRITION: Calories: 298 Cal Fat: 20 g Carbs: 4 g Protein: 8 g Fiber: 3 g

106. Salmon Salad with Feta Cheese

Preparation Time: 10'

Servings: 2

Cooking Time: 10'

Ingredients

- 10 ounces' salmon fillet, wild-caught
- 8 cherry tomatoes, diced
- ½ head of Romaine lettuce, cut into bite-sized pieces
- 1-ounce Kalamata olives
- 4 ounces' cucumber, diced
- 2 tablespoons mint, chopped
- ¼ of a medium red onion, peeled and sliced
- 1/3 teaspoon salt
- ¼ teaspoon ground black pepper
- 1 tablespoon lemon juice
- 1 tablespoon avocado oil
- 4 ounces' feta cheese, full-fat, crumbled
- Dressing
- ½ of lemon, juiced
- 1 medium avocado, peeled and pitted
- ¼ teaspoon salt
- ¼ teaspoon ground black pepper
- ½ teaspoon minced garlic
- 2 tablespoons avocado oil

Directions

1. Take a griddle pan, place it over medium-high heat, add oil, and let it heat.
2. Season salmon with salt and black pepper, place it on the heated pan, and cook for 4–5 minutes per side until seared.
3. Meanwhile, take a large salad bowl, place in it the remaining ingredients for the salad, and toss until mixed.
4. Prepare the dressing and for this, place all of its ingredients in a blender and pulse until smooth.
5. When salmon has cooked, transfer it to a cutting board, cool for 5 minutes, and cut it into slices.
6. Arrange salmon slices over the salad, drizzle with the salad dressing, and then serve.

Nutrition: Calories: 138 Cal Fat: 21 g Carbs: 5 g Protein: 9 g Fiber: 2 g

107. Spicy Shrimp Salad

PREPARATION TIME:	10'		SERVINGS:	2

COOKING TIME:	8'

INGREDIENTS

- 10 ounces' shrimps, peeled and deveined
- 2 medium avocados; peeled, pitted, diced
- ½ teaspoon minced garlic
- 5 ounces' cucumber, peeled and sliced
- ½ of a lime, juiced
- 2 ounces' baby spinach
- 2/3 teaspoon salt
- 2 teaspoons red chili powder
- ¼ teaspoon ground black pepper
- 3 tablespoons avocado oil
- Dressing
- ½ teaspoon minced garlic
- 1 tablespoon ginger, grated
- ¼ teaspoon salt
- ¼ teaspoon ground black pepper
- ½ of a lime, juiced
- ½ tablespoon soy sauce
- ¼ cup avocado oil

DIRECTIONS

1. Take a medium-sized bowl, place avocado slices in it, and drizzle with one-fourth of the lime juice.
2. Take a shallow dish or a plate, place avocado slices in it, add cucumber and spinach, sprinkle with 1/3 teaspoon salt, and toss until combined.
3. Take a large frying pan, place it over medium heat, add oil, and when hot, add garlic and red chili powder and cook for 1 minute until beginning to turn golden-brown.
4. Add shrimps, cook for 2–3 minutes until pink, flip the shrimps, and continue cooking for another 2–3 minutes until cooked.
5. When done, transfer shrimps to a plate, season with remaining salt and black pepper, and arrange them on top of the vegetables.
6. Prepare the dressing, and for this, place all of its ingredients in the blender, pulse until well combined, and then drizzle over the salad.
7. Serve straight away.

NUTRITION: Calories: 201 Cal Fat: 21 g Carbs: 5 g Protein: 5 g Fiber: 2 g

108. Keto Mustard Salad

Preparation Time: 15'		**Servings:** 2
	Cooking Time: 0'	

Ingredients

- ½ pound green cabbage, cored and shredded
- ½ of a lemon, juiced
- 1 tablespoon Dijon mustard
- 1/8 teaspoon fennel seeds
- 1 teaspoon salt
- 1/8 teaspoon ground black pepper
- ½ cup mayonnaise, full-fat

Directions

1. Take a medium-sized bowl, place shredded cabbage in it, sprinkle with salt, and drizzle with lemon juice.
2. Toss until combined and then let the cabbage rest for 10 minutes until slightly wilted.
3. Drain the cabbage, add mustard, salt, black pepper, fennel seeds, and mayonnaise, and stir until well mixed.

Nutrition: Calories: 209 Cal Fat: 21 g Carbs: 4 g Protein: 8 g Fiber: 3 g

109. WARM KALE SALAD

PREPARATION TIME:	10'		SERVINGS:	4

	COOKING TIME:	5'

INGREDIENTS

- 8 ounces' kale, destemmed and cut into small pieces
- ½ teaspoon minced garlic
- 1/3 teaspoon salt
- ¼ teaspoon ground black pepper
- 1 teaspoon Dijon mustard
- 2 tablespoons avocado oil
- 2 tablespoons mayonnaise, full-fat
- 2 ounces unsalted butter
- ¾ cup heavy whipping cream, full-fat
- 4 ounces' feta cheese, full-fat

DIRECTIONS

1. Prepare the dressing and for this, take a medium-sized bowl, pour in oil, cream, mayonnaise; add mustard, garlic, salt, and black pepper. Whisk until well combined and set aside until needed.
2. Take a large frying pan, place it over medium heat, add butter, and when it melts, add kale leaves.
3. Toss until coated, cook for 3 minutes, and season with salt and black pepper.
4. Transfer kale to the bowl, pour the prepared dressing over the kale, and stir until mixed.
5. Top feta cheese over kale and then serve.

NUTRITION: Calories: 488 Cal Fat: 27 g Carbs: 4 g Protein: 8 g Fiber: 3 g

110. Broccoli Salad with Dill

| PREPARATION TIME: | 15' | | SERVINGS: | 4 |

| COOKING TIME: | 10' |

INGREDIENTS

- 1 pound head of broccoli
- 4 slices of bacon, cooked and crumbled
- 1/3 teaspoon salt
- ¾ cup dill, fresh
- ¼ teaspoon ground black pepper
- 1 cup mayonnaise, full-fat

DIRECTIONS

1. Prepare the broccoli and for this, cut its florets and stem into very small pieces.
2. Take a large pot half full with salty water, place it over medium-high heat, and bring it to a boil.
3. Add broccoli florets and stems into the boiling water, boil for 5 minutes (or more, until fork-tender but crisp), and drain.
4. Place broccoli florets and stem into a large bowl and let it cool for 10 minutes.
5. Add remaining ingredients and stir until mixed.
6. Serve straight away.

NUTRITION: Calories: 418 Cal Fat: 12 g Carbs: 5 g Protein: 9g Fiber: 3 g

111. Collagen Mug Cake

Preparation Time: 5'

Servings: 1

Cooking Time: 2'

Ingredients

- 2 eggs, pasteurized, at room temperature
- 1 scoop of keto collagen
- ¼ teaspoon of sea salt
- ½ teaspoon baking powder
- 1 tablespoon cacao powder, unsweetened
- 10 drops of liquid stevia
- 1 tablespoon sunflower butter
- 1 teaspoon clarified butter
- 2 tablespoons coconut milk, full-fat

Directions

1. Take a large microwave-proof mug, crack eggs in it, add sunflower butter and milk, and whisk until blended.
2. Add cacao powder, salt, and baking powder, stir until combined, and whisk in collagen until smooth.
3. Place the mug into the microwave and cook for 2 minutes on high heat until done.
4. When done, drizzle clarified butter over the cake and then serve.

Nutrition: Calories: 418 Cal Fat: 10 g Carbs: 4 g Protein: 27 g Fiber: 3 g

112. Chocolate and Nut Butter Cups

Preparation Time: 35'

Servings: 6

Cooking Time: 2'

Ingredients

- 1-ounce chocolate, unsweetened
- 1/3 cup stevia
- 1 stick of unsalted butter
- 4 tablespoons peanut butter
- 2 tablespoons heavy cream

Directions

1. Take a medium-sized bowl, place unsalted butter in it, and then microwave for 1–2 minutes until butter melts, stirring every 30 seconds.
2. Add stevia, peanut butter, and cream, and then stir until combined.
3. Take a muffin tray, line six cups with a cupcake liner, fill them evenly with chocolate mixture, and freeze for a minimum of 30 minutes until firm.
4. Serve straight away.

Nutrition: Calories: 120 Cal Fat: 17 g Carbs: 5 g Protein: 9 g Fiber: 12 g

113. Peanut Butter Cup Chaffle

| PREPARATION TIME: | 10' | | SERVINGS: | 4 |

| COOKING TIME: | 20' |

INGREDIENTS

Chaffle:
- 2 teaspoons coconut flour
- 2 tablespoons cocoa powder, unsweetened
- ½ teaspoon baking powder
- 2 tablespoons swerve sweetener
- 1 teaspoon vanilla extract, unsweetened
- 1 teaspoon cake batter extract, unsweetened
- 4 tablespoons heavy cream, full-fat
- 4 eggs, pasteurized, at room temperature

Filling:
- 4 teaspoons erythritol sweetener
- 6 tablespoons peanut butter
- 4 tablespoons heavy cream, full-fat

DIRECTIONS

1. Switch on the waffle maker and set it to preheat according to the manufacturer's instructions.
2. Meanwhile, prepare the batter and for this, take a medium-sized bowl, add all the ingredients to it, and whisk well by using an electric mixer at medium speed until incorporated and smooth batter comes together.
3. Grease the waffle maker with avocado oil spray and ladle the prepared batter on waffle trays.
4. Shut the waffle maker with its lid and let cook for 5–8 minutes until waffle turns firm and golden-brown.
5. When done, remove waffles by using a tong or a fork and repeat with the remaining batter.
6. While chaffle cooks, prepare the filling, and for this, take a medium-sized bowl, place all of its ingredients in it, and whisk until combined.
7. Let waffles cool slightly, spread the prepared filling on top, sandwich two chaffles together, and serve.

NUTRITION: Calories: 128 Cal Fat: 17 g Carbs: 4 g Protein: 9g Fiber: 3 g

114. Cinnamon Sugar Chaffle

Preparation Time: 10'

Cooking Time: 20'

Servings: 4

Ingredients

- 8 tablespoons almond flour
- 2 teaspoons ground cinnamon
- 8 tablespoons erythritol sweeteners
- 1 teaspoon baking powder
- 4 teaspoons vanilla extract, unsweetened
- 4 tablespoons sour cream, full-fat
- 1 cup mozzarella cheese, full-fat, shredded
- 4 eggs, pasteurized, at room temperature

Directions

1. Switch on the waffle maker and set it to preheat according to the manufacturer's instructions.
2. Meanwhile, prepare the batter and for this, take a medium-sized bowl, add all the ingredients (except for cheese), whisk well until incorporated, and fold in cheese until combined.
3. Grease the waffle maker with avocado oil spray and ladle the prepared batter on waffle trays.
4. Shut the waffle maker with its lid and let cook for 5–8 minutes until waffle turns firm and golden-brown.
5. When done, remove waffles by using a tong or a fork and repeat with the remaining batter.
6. Let waffles cool slightly and serve

Nutrition: Calories: 267 Cal Fat: 10 g Carbs: 4 g Protein: 8 g Fiber: 3 g

115. Cinnamon and Cream Cheese Chaffle

Preparation Time:	10'	**Servings:**	4

Cooking Time: 20'

Ingredients

- 4 tablespoons almond flour
- 2 tablespoons erythritol sweetener
- 2 teaspoons ground cinnamon
- 1 teaspoon baking powder
- 2 tablespoons whey protein powder, unflavored
- ½ teaspoon vanilla extract, unsweetened
- 2 eggs, pasteurized, at room temperature
- ½ cup cream cheese, full-fat, softened

Directions

1. Switch on the waffle maker and set it to preheat according to the manufacturer's instructions.
2. Meanwhile, prepare the batter and for this, take a medium-sized bowl, crack eggs in it, add cinnamon and sweetener, and whisk well by using an electric mixer at medium speed until fluffy.
3. Add remaining ingredients and whisk until incorporated and smooth batter comes together.
4. Grease the waffle maker with avocado oil spray and ladle the prepared batter on waffle trays.
5. Shut the waffle maker with its lid and let cook for 5–8 minutes until waffle turns firm and golden-brown.
6. When done, remove waffles by using a tong or a fork and repeat with the remaining batter.
7. Let waffles cool slightly and serve.

Nutrition: Calories: 225 Cal Fat: 22 g Carbs: 6 g Protein: 4 g Fiber: 8 g

116. Golden Chaffles

Preparation Time: 10'

Cooking Time: 20'

Servings: 4

Ingredients

- 6 tablespoons almond flour
- 1 ½ teaspoon baking powder
- 1 tablespoon erythritol sweetener
- 1 teaspoon vanilla extract, unsweetened
- 4 eggs, pasteurized, at room temperature
- 2 1/3 cups mozzarella cheese, full-fat, shredded

Directions

1. Switch on the waffle maker and set it to preheat according to the manufacturer's instructions.
2. Meanwhile, prepare the batter and for this, take a medium-sized bowl, place flour in it, add baking powder and sweetener, and stir until combined.
3. Then add vanilla, cheese, and eggs, and whisk well by using an electric mixer at medium speed until incorporated and smooth batter comes together.
4. Grease the waffle maker with avocado oil spray and ladle the prepared batter on waffle trays.
5. Shut the waffle maker with its lid and then let cook for 5–8 minutes until the waffle turns firm and golden-brown.
6. When done, remove waffles by using a tong or a fork and repeat with the remaining batter.
7. Let waffles cool slightly and serve.

Nutrition: Calories: 168 Cal Fat: 10 g Carbs: 2 g Protein: 4 g Fiber: 3 g

117. Churro Chaffle

Preparation Time: 10'

Servings: 4

Cooking Time: 20'

Ingredients

Chaffle:
- 8 teaspoons coconut flour
- 4 teaspoons pumpkin pie spice
- 8 tablespoons swerve sweetener
- 1 teaspoon baking powder
- 2 teaspoons vanilla extract, unsweetened
- 4 eggs, pasteurized, at room temperature
- 4 tablespoons unsalted butter, melted
- 2 cups mozzarella cheese, full-fat, shredded

Topping:
- 2 2/3 teaspoons ground cinnamon
- 1 cup swerve sweetener
- 1 1/3 teaspoons ground nutmeg
- 8 tablespoons unsalted butter, melted

Directions

1. Switch on the waffle maker and set it to preheat according to the manufacturer's instructions.
2. Meanwhile, prepare the batter and for this, take a medium-sized bowl, add all the ingredients to it, and whisk well by using an electric mixer at medium speed until incorporated and smooth batter comes together.
3. Grease the waffle maker with avocado oil spray and ladle the prepared batter on waffle trays.
4. Shut the waffle maker with its lid and let cook for 5–8 minutes until waffle turns firm and golden-brown.
5. When done, remove waffles by using a tong or a fork and repeat with the remaining batter.
6. While Chaffle cooks, prepare the topping, and for this, take a medium-sized bowl, place cinnamon, sweetener, and nutmeg, and stir until mixed.
7. Let waffles cool slightly, brush with butter, sprinkle cinnamon mixture on top, and serve.

Nutrition: Calories: 212 Cal Fat: 19 g Carbs: 5 g Protein: 4 g Fiber: 2 g

KETO DIET COOKBOOK *for women over 50*

118. Yogurt Chaffle

Preparation Time: 10'

Servings: 4

Cooking Time: 20'

Ingredients

- 2 cups mozzarella cheese, full-fat, shredded
- 4 eggs, pasteurized, at room temperature
- 8 tablespoons ground almonds
- 2 teaspoons psyllium husk
- 2 teaspoons baking powder
- 4 tablespoons yogurt, full-fat

Directions

1. Switch on the waffle maker and set it to preheat according to the manufacturer's instructions.
2. Meanwhile, prepare the batter and for this, take a medium-sized bowl, add all the ingredients, whisk well by using an electric mixer at medium speed until incorporated, and let the mixture sit for 5 minutes.
3. Grease the waffle maker with avocado oil spray and ladle the prepared batter on waffle trays.
4. Shut the waffle maker with its lid and let cook for 5–8 minutes until waffle turns firm and golden-brown.
5. When done, remove waffles by using a tong or a fork and repeat with the remaining batter.
6. Let waffles cool slightly and serve.

Nutrition: Calories: 131 Cal Fat: 6 g Carbs: 3 g Protein: 9 g Fiber: 3 g

119. Zucchini Chaffle

PREPARATION TIME: 10'	**SERVINGS:** 4

COOKING TIME: 20'

INGREDIENTS

- 2 cups zucchini, grated
- 1 ½ teaspoon salt, divided
- 1 teaspoon ground black pepper
- 2 teaspoons dried basil
- 1 cup parmesan cheese, full-fat, shredded
- 2 eggs, pasteurized, at room temperature
- ½ cup mozzarella cheese, shredded

DIRECTIONS

1. Place grated zucchini in a colander, sprinkle with ¼ teaspoon salt, toss until mixed, and then let it sit for 5 minutes.
2. Meanwhile, switch on the waffle maker and set it to preheat according to the manufacturer's instructions.
3. After 5 minutes, wrap grated zucchini in a paper towel and press tightly to squeeze out moisture as much as possible.
4. Meanwhile, prepare the batter and for this, take a medium-sized bowl, crack the eggs in it, and whisk until blended.
5. Add zucchini in it along with remaining salt, black pepper, basil, and mozzarella cheese, and stir until mixed.
6. Grease the waffle maker with avocado oil spray, sprinkle 2 tablespoons of parmesan cheese on waffle trays until covered, and ladle the prepared batter on top.
7. Top batter with another 2 tablespoons of parmesan cheese, shut the waffle maker with its lid, and let cook for 5–8 minutes until waffle turns firm and golden-brown.
8. When done, remove waffles by using a tong or a fork and repeat with the remaining batter and parmesan cheese.
9. Let waffles cool slightly and serve

NUTRITION: Calories: 128 Cal Fat: 9 g Carbs: 7 g Protein: 8 g Fiber: 5 g

120. Cauliflower Chaffle

PREPARATION TIME: 10'

SERVINGS: 4

COOKING TIME: 20'

INGREDIENTS

- 2 cups cauliflower florets, grated
- ½ teaspoon garlic powder
- ½ teaspoon salt
- ½ teaspoon ground black pepper
- 1 teaspoon Italian seasoning
- 2 eggs, pasteurized, at room temperature
- 1 cup mozzarella cheese, full-fat, shredded
- 1 cup parmesan cheese, full-fat, shredded

DIRECTIONS

1. Switch on the waffle maker and set it to preheat according to the manufacturer's instructions.
2. Meanwhile, prepare the batter and for this, take a medium-sized bowl, add all the ingredients to it, and whisk well by using an electric mixer at medium speed until incorporated and smooth batter comes together.
3. Grease the waffle maker with avocado oil spray, sprinkle 2 tablespoons of parmesan cheese on waffle trays until covered, and ladle the prepared batter on top.
4. Shut the waffle maker with its lid and let cook for 5–8 minutes until waffle turns firm and golden-brown.
5. When done, remove waffles by using a tong or a fork and repeat with the remaining batter.
6. Let waffles cool slightly and serve.

NUTRITION: Calories: 290 Cal Fat: 13 g Carbs: 5 g Protein: 9 g Fiber: 4 g

121. Zesty Chili Lime Tuna Salad

Preparation Time: 10'	**Servings:** 4
Cooking Time: 0'	

Ingredients

- 1 tablespoon of lime juice
- 1/3 cup of mayonnaise
- ¼ teaspoon of salt
- 1 teaspoon of Tajin chili lime seasoning
- 1/8 teaspoon of pepper
- 1 medium stalk celery (finely chopped)
- 2 cups of romaine lettuce (chopped roughly)
- 2 tablespoons of red onion (finely chopped)
- optional: chopped green onion, black pepper, lemon juice
- 5 ozs. canned tuna

Directions

1. Using a bowl of medium size, mix some of the ingredients such as lime, pepper and chili lime
2. Then, add tuna and vegetables to the pot and stir. You can serve with cucumber, celery or a bed of greens

Nutrition: Calories:409 Cal Fat: 37 g Carbs: 4 g Protein: 9 g Fiber: 3 g

122. Sheet Pan Brussels Sprouts and Bacon

Preparation Time: 5'

Servings: 4

Cooking Time: 35'

Ingredients

- 6 ozs. bacon
- 6 ozs. raw brussels sprouts
- Salt
- Pepper

Directions

1. Prepare the oven by preheating it to 400 degrees, Then, prepare the baking sheet with parchment paper
2. Prepare brussels sprouts in the pan
3. Use kitchen shears to cut the bacon into little pieces
4. Add the cut bacon and brussels sprouts into the baking sheet already prepared. Then, add pepper and salt
5. Bake for up to 45 minutes. Allow the Brussel sprouts to become crispy

Nutrition: Calories: 138 Cal Fat: 20 g Carbs: 6 g Protein: 7 g Fiber: 4 g

123. Super Simple Chicken Cauliflower Fried Rice

| PREPARATION TIME: | 5′ | | SERVINGS: | 4 |

| COOKING TIME: | 20′ |

INGREDIENTS

- ½ teaspoon of sesame oil
- 1 small carrot (chopped)
- 1 tablespoon of avocado or coconut oil
- 1 small onion (finely sliced)
- ½ cup of snap peas (chopped)
- ½ cup of red peppers cut finely
- 1 tablespoon of garlic
- 1 tablespoon of garlic, properly chopped
- 1 teaspoon of salt
- 2 teaspoons of garlic powder
- 4 chicken breasts, chopped and cooked
- 4 cups of rice cauliflower
- 2 large scrambled eggs
- Gluten-free soy sauce, one quarter cup size

DIRECTIONS

1. Gently season the chicken breasts with ½ tablespoon of salt, ¼ tablespoon of pepper, and ½ tablespoon of olive oil. Cook the chicken on any pan of your choice
2. Add coconut/olive/avocado oil. Cut some onions and carrots and sauce and leave for up to 3 minutes
3. Next, add the rest of the vegetables, pepper/salt/garlic powder and then cook for extra 3 minutes
4. Put in fresh garlic coconut aminos or soy sauce and riced cauliflower; then stir
5. Add scrambled eggs and chicken and mix until they are well combined
6. Put off the heat and then stir in some green peas. Season again, you can top it with sesame seeds if you like

NUTRITION: Calories: 260 Cal Fat: 21 g Carbs: 6 g Protein: 3 g Fiber: 4 g

124. Prep-Ahead Low-Carb Casserole

PREPARATION TIME: 5'

SERVINGS: 4

COOKING TIME: 35'

INGREDIENTS

- 1 cooked and cubed chicken breast
- 4 cooked and crumbled strips of bacon
- ½ cup of celery, chopped
- 1/3 cup of mozzarella cheese
- 1 tablespoon of Italian seasoning
- ½ cup of grated parmesan
- 3 whisked eggs
- ¼ whipping cream

DIRECTIONS

1. Start by pre-heating the oven to at least above 350 degrees °F. Use a non-stick cooking spray to spray a casserole dish
2. Combine all the ingredients, leaving out the only mozzarella with a mixing bowl. Continue mixing until properly combined
3. Pour out the mixture into a casserole dish. You can top it with mozzarella
4. Bake for up to 35 minutes. Then, increase the heat and allow to boil until the mozzarella turns to golden brown
5. Allow it to cool before serving

NUTRITION: Calories: 234 Cal Fat: 20 g Carbs: 3 g Protein: 9 g Fiber: 2 g

125. BBQ Pulled Beef Sando

Preparation Time: 5'

Servings: 4

Cooking Time: 10-12 hours

Ingredients

- 3 lbs. boneless chuck roasts
- 2 tablespoons of pink Himalayan salt
- 2 tablespoons of garlic powder
- 1 tablespoon of onion powder
- ¼ apple cider vinegar
- 2 tablespoons of coconut aminos
- ½ cup of bone broth
- ¼ cup of melted Kerry gold butter
- 1 tablespoon of black pepper
- 1 tablespoon of smoked paprika
- 2 tablespoons of tomato paste

Directions

1. Trim the fat from the beef and slice it into two huge pieces
2. Mix salt, onion, paprika, black pepper, and garlic. Next is to rub the mixture on the beef and then put the beef in a slow cooker
3. Use another bowl to melt butter. Then, add a tomato paste, coconut aminos, and vinegar. Pour it all over the beef. Next is to add the bone broth into the slow cooker by pouring it around the beef
4. Cook for about 10 minutes. After that, take out the beef and increase the temperature of the cooker so that the sauce can thicken. Tear the beef before adding it to the slow cooker and toss with the sauce

Nutrition: Calories: 184 Cal Fat: 29 g Carbs: 7 g Protein: 11 g Fiber: 2 g

126. Keto-friendly Oatmeal Recipe

Preparation Time: 5'

Servings: 4

Cooking Time: 15'

Ingredients

- 1 tablespoon of flaxseed meal
- ½ cup of hemp hearts
- 1 tablespoon of chia seeds
- 1 tablespoon coconut flakes
- 1 cup of unsweetened almond milk
- 1 scoop of Vanilla MCT oil powder (1 tablespoon of coconut oil and 1 tablespoon of stevia)
- 1 teaspoon of cinnamon

Directions

1. Add all the ingredients in a saucepot and mix
2. Stir until it simmers and is thick enough to your liking
3. You can serve garnished with frozen berries

Nutrition: Calories: 189 Cal Fat: 22 g Carbs: 4 g Protein: 9 g Fiber: 5 g

127. CRUNCHY COCONUT CLUSTER KETO CEREAL

PREPARATION TIME: 5'		SERVINGS: 4
	COOKING TIME: 20'	

INGREDIENTS

- ½ cup of unsweetened shredded coconut
- ½ cup of hemp hearts
- ½ cup of raw pumpkin seeds
- A pinch of sea salt
- 2 scoops of perfect Keto MCT oil powder
- 1 white egg
- 1 teaspoon of cinnamon

DIRECTIONS

1. The oven should be pre-heated to 350o F
2. A sheet pan should then be lined with parchment paper
3. Stir all the dry ingredients in the bowl
4. Using a separate bowl, mix the white egg until it becomes frothy. Then, pour it slowly into the dry; mix
5. Transfer the mixture into a sheet of the pan and flatten to a thickness of ¼ of an inch
6. Leave to bake for 15 minutes. After removal, use a spatula to break up the mass into chunks and allow to bake for more 5 minutes
7. Finally, take it out of the oven and serve with your milk of choice. It can be stored for three days in an airtight container at room temperature

NUTRITION: Calories: 5258 Cal Fat: 25 g Carbs: 7 g Protein: 9 g Fiber: 2 g

128. Avocado Egg Bowls

PREPARATION TIME: 5'

SERVINGS: 4

COOKING TIME: 15'

INGREDIENTS

- 1 avocado halved with the removed stone
- 1 tablespoon of salted butter
- 3 free-range eggs
- 3 rashers of bacon into little pieces
- Black pepper and pinch of salt

DIRECTIONS

1. Begin by removing most of the avocado flesh, remaining just ½ inch on the avocado
2. Put in butter into a large saucepan while it's heating. Let the butter melt in the pan. Crack the eggs and beat them in a jug, adding a little pepper and salt
3. Put the bacon on one side of the pan and leave everything to fry for some minutes. Next, add the eggs to the opposite bottom of the pan and continue to stir until it is scrambled. The bacon and the eggs should be ready soon enough in 5 minutes. In case the scrambled eggs are done before the bacon, take it from the pan into a bowl
4. Mix the pieces of the bacon and the scrambled eggs in the pot and add into the avocado bowls

NUTRITION: Calories: 500 Cal Fat: 26 g Carbs: 6 g Protein: 9 g Fiber: 9 g

129. Keto Cinnamon Coffee

Preparation Time: 5'

Servings: 1

Cooking Time: 5'

Ingredients

- 2 tbsps. ground coffee
- 1/3 cup of heavy whipping cream
- 1 tsp. ground cinnamon
- 2 cups water

Directions

1. Start by mixing the cinnamon with the ground coffee.
2. Pour in hot water and do what you usually do when brewing. Use a mixer or whisk to whip the cream 'til you get stiff peaks Serve in a tall mug and put the whipped cream on the surface. Sprinkle with some cinnamon and enjoy.

Nutrition: Calories: 168 Cal Fat: 18 g Carbs: 7 g Protein: 9 g Fiber: 3 g

130. Keto Waffles and Blueberries

| PREPARATION TIME: | 5' | | SERVINGS: | 8 |

| COOKING TIME: | 15' |

INGREDIENTS

- 8 eggs
- 5 ozs. melted butter
- 1 tsp. vanilla extract
- 2 tsps. baking powder
- 1/3 cup coconut flour
- 3 ozs. butter (topping)
- 1 oz. fresh blueberries (topping)

DIRECTIONS

1. Start by mixing the butter and eggs first until you get a smooth batter. Put in the remaining ingredients except those that we'll be using as topping.
2. Heat your waffle iron to medium temperature and start pouring in the batter for cooking
3. In a separate bowl, mix the butter and blueberries using a hand mixer. Use this to top off your freshly cooked waffles

NUTRITION: Calories: 504 Cal Fat: 21 g Carbs: 5 g Protein: 7 g Fiber: 4 g

131. Baked Avocado Eggs

Preparation Time: 5'

Servings: 4

Cooking Time: 30'

Ingredients

- Avocados
- 4 eggs
- ½ cup of bacon bits, around 55 grams
- 2 tbsps. fresh chives, chopped
- 1 sprig of chopped fresh basil, chopped
- 1 cherry tomato, quartered
- Salt and pepper to taste
- Shredded cheddar cheese

Directions

1. Start by preheating the oven to 400 degrees Fahrenheit
2. Slice the avocado and remove the pits. Put them on a baking sheet and crack some eggs onto the center hole of the avocado. If it's too small, just scoop out more of the flesh to make room. Salt and pepper to taste.
3. Top with bacon bits and bake for 15 minutes. Remove and sprinkle with herbs. Enjoy!

Nutrition: Calories: 271 Cal Fat: 18 g Carbs: 7 g Protein: 9 g Fiber: 3 g

132. Mushroom Omelet

Preparation Time: 5′

Servings: 1

Cooking Time: 5′

Ingredients

- 3 eggs, medium
- 1 oz. shredded cheese
- 1 oz. butter used for frying
- ¼ yellow onion, chopped
- 4 large sliced mushrooms
- Your favorite vegetables, optional
- Salt and pepper to taste

Directions

1. Crack and whisk the eggs in a bowl. Add some salt and pepper to taste.
2. Melt the butter in a pan using low heat. Put in the mushroom and onion, cooking the two until you get that amazing smell.
3. Pour the egg mix into the pan and allow it to cook on medium heat.
4. Allow the bottom part to cook before sprinkling the cheese on top of the still-raw portion of the egg.
5. Carefully pry the edges of the omelet and fold it in half. Allow it to cook for a few more seconds before removing the pan from the heat and sliding it directly onto your plate.

Nutrition: Calories: 528 Cal Fat: 25g Carbs: 8 g Protein: 11 g Fiber: 3 g

133. CHOCOLATE SEA SALT SMOOTHIE

PREPARATION TIME: 5'

SERVINGS: 2

COOKING TIME: 5'

INGREDIENTS

- 1 avocado (frozen or not)
- 2 cups of almond milk
- 1 tbsp. tahini
- ¼ cup of cocoa powder
- 1 scoop Perfect Keto chocolate base

DIRECTIONS

1. Combine all the ingredients in a high-speed blender and mix until you get a soft smoothie.

NUTRITION: Calories: 238 Cal Fat: 19 g Carbs: 3 g Protein: 14 g Fiber: 3 g

134. Zucchini Lasagna

| PREPARATION TIME: | 20' | | SERVINGS: | 9 |

| COOKING TIME: | 80' |

INGREDIENTS

- 3 cups raw macadamia nuts or soaked blanched almonds (for ricotta)
- 2 tbsps. nutritional yeast (for ricotta)
- 2 tsps. dried oregano (for ricotta)
- 1 tsp. sea salt (for ricotta)
- 1/2 cup water or more as needed (for ricotta)
- 1/4 cup vegan parmesan cheese (for ricotta)
- 1 cup fresh basil, chopped (for ricotta)
- 1 medium lemon, juiced (for ricotta)
- Black pepper to taste (for ricotta)
- 1 28-oz. jar favorite marinara sauce
- 3 medium zucchinis squash thinly sliced with a mandolin

DIRECTIONS

1. Preheat the oven to 375 degrees Fahrenheit Put macadamia nuts to a food processor.
2. Add the remaining ingredients and continue to puree the mixture. You want to create a fine paste.
3. Taste and adjust the seasonings depending on your personal preferences.
4. Pour 1 cup of marinara sauce in a baking dish.
5. Start creating the lasagna layers using thinly sliced zucchini
6. Scoop small amounts of ricotta mixture on the zucchini and spread it into a thin layer. Continue the layering until you've run out of zucchini or space for it.
7. Sprinkle parmesan cheese on the topmost layer.
8. Cover the pan with foil and bake for 45 minutes. Remove the foil and bake for 15 minutes more.
9. Allow it to cool for 15 minutes before serving. Serve immediately. The lasagna will keep for 3 days in the fridge.

NUTRITION: Calories: 388 Cal Fat: 29 g Carbs: 9 g Protein: 10 g Fiber: 3 g

135. Vegan Keto Scramble

Preparation Time: 15'	**Servings:** 2
Cooking Time: 10'	

Ingredients

- 14 ozs. firm tofu
- 3 tbsps. avocado oil
- 2 tbsps. yellow onion, diced
- 1.5 tbsp. nutritional yeast
- ½ tsp. turmeric
- ½ tsp. garlic powder
- ½ tsp. salt
- 1 cup baby spinach
- 3 grape tomatoes
- 3 ozs. vegan cheddar cheese

Directions

1. Start by squeezing the water out of the tofu block using a clean cloth or a paper towel.
2. Grab a skillet and put it on medium heat. Sauté the chopped onion in a small amount of avocado oil until it starts to caramelize
3. Using a potato masher, crumble the tofu on the skillet. Do this thoroughly until the tofu looks a lot like scrambled eggs.
4. Drizzle some more of the avocado oil onto the mix together with the dry seasonings. Stir thoroughly and evenly distribute the flavor.
5. Cook under medium heat, occasionally stirring to avoid burning of the tofu. You'd want most of the liquid to evaporate until you get a nice chunk of scrambled tofu. Fold the baby spinach, cheese, and diced tomato. Cook for a few more minutes until the cheese melted. Serve and enjoy!

Nutrition: Calories: 208 Cal Fat: 19 g Carbs: 9 g Protein: 10 g Fiber: 5 g

136. Parmesan Cheese Strips

Preparation Time: 20'	Servings: 12

Cooking Time: 7'

Ingredients

- 1 cup shredded parmesan cheese
- 1 tsp dried basil

Directions

1. Preheat the oven to 350 degrees Fahrenheit. Prepare the baking sheet by lining it with parchment paper.
2. Form small piles of the parmesan cheese on the baking sheet. Flatten it out evenly and then sprinkle dried basil on top of the cheese.
3. Bake for 5 to 7 minutes or until you get a golden-brown color with crispy edges. Take it out, serve, and enjoy!

Nutrition: Calories: 90 Cal Fat: 18 g Carbs: 7 g Protein: 9 g Fiber: 3 g

137. Peanut Butter Power Granola

Preparation Time: 5′

Servings: 12

Cooking Time: 30′

Ingredients

- 1 cup shredded coconut or almond flour
- 1 1/2 cups almonds
- 1 1/2 cups pecans
- 1/3 cup swerve sweetener
- 1/3 cup vanilla whey protein, powder
- 1/3 cup peanut butter
- 1/4 cup sunflower seeds 1/4 cup butter
- 1/4 cup of water

Directions

1. Preheat the oven to 300 degrees Fahrenheit and prepare a baking sheet with parchment paper
2. Place the almonds and pecans in a food processor. Put them all in a large bowl and add the sunflower seeds, shredded coconut, vanilla, sweetener, and protein powder.
3. Melt the peanut butter and butter together in the microwave. Mix the melted butter in the nut mixture and stir it thoroughly until the nuts are well-distributed.
4. Put in the water to create a lumpy mixture. Scoop out small amounts of the mixture and place it on the baking sheet.
5. Bake for 30 minutes. Enjoy!

Nutrition: Calories: 168 Cal Fat: 18 g Carbs: 7 g Protein: 9 g Fiber: 3 g

138. Homemade Graham Crackers

Preparation Time:	5′		Servings:	10

	Cooking Time:	30′

Ingredients

- 1 egg, large
- 2 cups almond flour
- 1/3 cup swerve brown
- 2 tsps. cinnamon
- 1 tsp. baking powder
- 2 tbsps. melted butter
- 1 tsp. vanilla extract
- Salt

Directions

1. Preheat the oven to 300 degrees Fahrenheit
2. Grab a bowl and whisk the almond flour, cinnamon, sweetener, baking powder, and salt. Stir all the ingredients together.
3. Put in the egg, molasses, melted butter, and vanilla extract. Stir until you get a dough-like consistency.
4. Roll out the dough evenly, making sure that you don't go beyond ¼ of an inch thick. Cut the dough into the shapes you want for cooking. Transfer it on the baking tray
5. Bake for 20 to 30 minutes until it firms up. Let it cool for 30 minutes outside of the oven and then put them back in for another 30 minutes. Make sure that for the second time putting the biscuit, the temperature is not higher than 200 degrees Fahrenheit. This last step will make the biscuit crispy.

Nutrition: Calories: 158 Cal Fat: 21 g Carbs: 8 g Protein: 8 g Fiber: 3 g

139. KETO NO-BAKE COOKIES

PREPARATION TIME: 5′

SERVINGS: 18

COOKING TIME: 10′

INGREDIENTS

- 2/3 cup of all-natural peanut butter
- 1 cup of all-natural shredded coconut, unsweetened
- 2 tbsps. real butter
- 4 drops of vanilla

DIRECTIONS

1. Melt the butter in the microwave.
2. Take it out and put it in the peanut butter. Stir thoroughly. Add the sweetener and coconut. Mix.
3. Spoon it onto a pan lined with parchment paper Freeze for 10 minutes
4. Cut into preferred slices. Store in an airtight container in the fridge and enjoy whenever.

NUTRITION: Calories: 80 Cal Fat: 21 g Carbs: 8 g Protein: 10 g Fiber: 3 g

140. Swiss Cheese Crunchy Nachos

PREPARATION TIME: 5′

SERVINGS: 2

COOKING TIME: 15′

INGREDIENTS

- ½ cup shredded Swiss cheese
- ½ cup shredded cheddar cheese
- 1/8 cup cooked bacon pieces

DIRECTIONS

1. Preheat the oven to 300 degrees Fahrenheit and prepare the baking sheet by lining it with parchment paper.
2. Start by spreading the Swiss cheese on the parchment. Sprinkle it with bacon and then top it off again with the cheese.
3. Bake until the cheese has melted. This should take around 10 minutes or less.
4. Allow the cheese to cool before cutting them into triangle strips.
5. Grab another baking sheet and place the triangle cheese strips on top.
6. Broil them for 2 to 3 minutes so they'll get chunky.

NUTRITION: Calories: 280 Cal Fat: 21 g Carbs: 5 g Protein: 9 g Fiber: 3 g

141. Keto Cheesecake with Blueberries

Preparation Time:	5'		Servings:	12

	Cooking Time:	90'	

Ingredients

- 1¼ cups almond flour (crust)
- 2 tbsps. erythritol (crust)
- ½ tsp of vanilla extract (crust)
- 2 ozs. butter (crust)
- 20 ozs. cream cheese (filling)
- 2 eggs (filling)
- ½ cup of Crème Fraîche or heavy whipping cream (filling)
- 1 tsp lemon zest (filling)
- ½ tsp of vanilla extract (filling)
- 2 ozs. fresh blueberries (optional)

Directions

1. Preheat the oven to 350 degrees Fahrenheit.
2. While waiting, prepare a spring form pan by lining it with butter or putting in parchment paper.
3. Melt the butter until you smell that nutty scent. This will help create a toffee flavor for the crust.
4. Remove the pan from the heat and add almond flour, vanilla, and sweetener. Mix the ingredients until you get a dough-like consistency.
5. Press it into the pan and bake for 8 minutes until you get a slightly golden crust. Set aside to cool.
6. Now we're going to work on the filling. Mix all the filling ingredients together and beat it heavily. Pour the mixture on the crust.
7. Increase the oven's heat to 400 degrees Fahrenheit and bake for the next 15 minutes.
8. Once done, lower it to 230 degrees Fahrenheit and bake again for 45 to 60 minutes
9. Turn the heat off and leave it inside in the oven to cool.
10. Remove after it has cooled completely. You can store it in the fridge and serve with fresh blueberries on top.

Nutrition: Calories: 288 Cal Fat: 33 g Carbs: 7 g Protein: 12 g Fiber: 3 g

142. Keto Lemon Ice Cream

Preparation Time: 5'		**Servings:** 10

Cooking Time: 90'

Ingredients

- 6 servings Ingredients:
- 3 eggs
- 1 lemon, zest, and juice
- 1/3 cup erythritol
- 1¾ cups heavy whipping cream

Directions

1. Grate the lemon to get the zest and then squeeze out the juice. Set it aside in the meantime.
2. Separate the eggs. Using a hand mixer beat the eggs until they become stiff. Afterward, beat the egg yolks and sweetener until it becomes light and fluffy.
3. Add the lemon juice in the egg yolks. Beat it before carefully folding the egg whites into the yolk.
4. In a separate bowl, whip the cream until you get a soft peak. Gently fold the egg mixture into the cream
5. Pour the whole thing into an ice cream maker and use it according to instructions of the manufacturer.
6. For those who don't have an ice cream maker, you can just put the bowl in the freezer. You'll have to take it out every 30 minutes to stir it. This should be done for the next two hours until you get the consistency you want.

Nutrition: Calories: 168 Cal Fat: 27 g Carbs: 7 g Protein: 9 g Fiber: 3 g

143. Peanut Butter Balls

Preparation Time: 5'	**Servings:** 18
Cooking Time: 20'	

Ingredients

- 1 cup of salted peanuts chopped finely (not peanut flour)
- 1 cup of peanut butter
- 1 cup of sweetener
- 8 ozs. of sugar-free chocolate chips

Directions

1. Mix the peanut butter, sweetener, and chopped peanuts together.
2. You'll get a dough-light substance by doing this.
3. Knead until smooth and then divide the dough into 18 pieces. Shape them into balls.
4. Place the dough on a baking sheet lined with wax paper before putting them in the fridge to harden.
5. In the meantime, melt the chocolate chips in a microwave.
6. Take out the peanut butter balls and dip them in the melted chocolate. Put them back in the fridge to set. Enjoy!

Nutrition: Calories: 194 Cal Fat: 18 g Carbs: 5 g Protein: 10 g Fiber: 5 g

144. Classic Pork Tenderloin

PREPARATION TIME:	15'		SERVINGS:	4

COOKING TIME: 35'

INGREDIENTS

- 8 bacon slices
- 2 lbs. pork tenderloin
- 1 tsp. dried oregano, crushed
- 1 tsp. dried basil, crushed
- 1 tbsp. garlic powder
- 1 tsp. seasoned salt
- 3 tbsps. butter

DIRECTIONS

1. Preheat the oven to 400 degrees F.
2. Heat a large ovenproof skillet over medium-high heat and cook the bacon for about 6-7 minutes.
3. Transfer the bacon onto a paper towel-lined plate to drain.
4. Then, wrap the pork tenderloin with bacon slices and secure with toothpicks.
5. With a sharp knife, slice the tenderloin between each bacon slice to make a medallion.
6. In a bowl, mix together the dried herbs, garlic powder, and seasoned salt.
7. Now, coat the medallion with herb mixture.
8. With a paper towel, wipe out the skillet.
9. In the same skillet, melt the butter over medium-high heat and cook the pork medallion for about 4 minutes per side.
10. Now, transfer the skillet into the oven.
11. Roast for about 17-20 minutes.
12. Remove the wok from oven and let it cool slightly before cutting.
13. Cut the tenderloin into desired size slices and serve.

NUTRITION: Calories: 471 Cal Fat: 19 g Carbs: 8 g Protein: 9 g Fiber: 3 g

145. Signature Italian Pork Dish

Preparation Time: 15′

Servings: 6

Cooking Time: 15′

Ingredients

- 2 lbs. pork tenderloins, cut into 1½-inch pieces
- ¼ cup of. almond flour
- 1 tsp. garlic salt
- Freshly ground black pepper, to taste
- 2 tbsps. butter
- ½ cup of homemade chicken broth
- 1/3 cup of balsamic vinegar
- 1 tbsp. capers
- 2 tsps. fresh lemon zest, grated finely

Directions

1. In a large bowl, add the pork pieces, flour, garlic salt, and black pepper and toss to coat well.
2. Remove pork pieces from the bowl and shake off excess flour mixture.
3. In a large skillet, melt the butter over medium-high heat and cook the pork pieces for about 2-3 minutes per side.
4. Add broth and vinegar and bring to a gentle boil.
5. Reduce the heat to medium and simmer for about 3-4 minutes.
6. With a slotted spoon, transfer the pork pieces onto a plate.
7. In the same skillet, add the capers and lemon zest and simmer for about 3-5 minutes or until desired thickness of the sauce.
8. Pour sauce over pork pieces and serve.

Nutrition: Calories: 484 Cal Fat: 19 g Carbs: 8 g Protein: 10 g Fiber: 5 g

146. FLAVOR PACKED PORK LOIN

PREPARATION TIME: 15'

SERVINGS: 6

COOKING TIME: 60'

INGREDIENTS

- 1/3 cup of low-sodium soy sauce
- ¼ cup of fresh lemon juice
- 2 tsps. fresh lemon zest, grated
- 1 tbsp. fresh thyme, finely chopped
- 2 tbsps. fresh ginger, grated
- 2 garlic cloves, chopped finely
- 2 tbsps. Erythritol
- Freshly ground black pepper, to taste
- ½ tsp. cayenne pepper
- 2 lbs. boneless pork loin

DIRECTIONS

1. For pork marinade: in a large baking dish, add all the ingredients except pork loin and mix until well combined.
2. Add the pork loin and coat with the marinade generously.
3. Refrigerate for about 24 hours.
4. Preheat the oven to 400 degrees F.
5. Remove the pork loin from marinade and arrange it into a baking dish.
6. Cover the baking dish and bake for about 1 hour.
7. Remove from the oven and place the pork loin onto a cutting board.
8. With a piece of foil, cover each loin for at least 10 minutes before slicing.
9. With a sharp knife, cut the pork loin into desired size slices and serve.

NUTRITION: Calories: 230 Cal Fat: 29 g Carbs: 4 g Protein: 10 g Fiber: 6 g

147. Spiced Pork Tenderloin

Preparation Time: 15'

Servings: 6

Cooking Time: 18'

Ingredients

- 2 tsps. fresh rosemary, minced
- 2 tsps. fennel seeds
- 2 tsps. coriander seeds
- 2 tsps. caraway seeds
- 1 tsps. cumin seeds
- 1 bay leaf
- Salt and freshly ground black pepper, to taste
- 2 tbsps. fresh dill, chopped
- 2 (1-lb.) pork tenderloins, trimmed

Directions

1. For the spice rub: in a spice grinder, add the seeds and bay leaf and grind until finely powdered.
2. Add the salt and black pepper and mix.
3. In a small bowl, reserve 2 tbsp. of spice rub.
4. In another small bowl, mix together the remaining spice rub, and dill.
5. Place 1 tenderloin over a piece of plastic wrap.
6. With a sharp knife, slice through the meat to within ½-inch of the opposite side. Now, open the tenderloin like a book. Cover with another plastic wrap and with a meat pounder, gently pound into ½-inch thickness. Repeat with the remaining tenderloin. Remove the plastic wrap and spread half of the dill mixture over the center of each tenderloin.
7. Roll each tenderloin like a cylinder.
8. With a kitchen string, tightly tie each roll at several places.
9. Rub each roll with the reserved spice rub generously.
10. With 1 plastic wrap, wrap each roll and refrigerate for at least 4-6 hours.
11. Preheat the grill to medium-high heat. Grease the grill grate.
12. Remove the plastic wrap from tenderloins.
13. Place tenderloins onto the grill and cook for about 14-18 minutes, flipping occasionally.
14. Remove from the grill and place tenderloins onto a cutting board and with a piece of foil, cover each tenderloin for at least 5-10 minutes before slicing.
15. With a sharp knife, cut the tenderloins into desired size slices and serve.

Nutrition: Calories: 309 Cal Fat: 30 g Carbs: 20 g Protein: 19 g Fiber: 9 g

148. Sticky Pork Ribs

PREPARATION TIME:	5'		SERVINGS:	9

COOKING TIME: 2 h 30'

Ingredients

- ¼ cup of erythritol
- 1 tbsp. garlic powder
- 1 tbsp. paprika
- ½ tsp. red chili powder
- 4 lbs. pork ribs, membrane removed
- Salt and freshly ground black pepper, to taste
- 1½ tsp. liquid smoke
- 1½ cup of sugar-free BBQ sauce

Directions

1. Preheat the oven to 300 degrees F. Line a large baking sheet with 2 layers of foil, shiny side out. In a bowl, add the Erythritol, garlic powder, paprika, and chili powder and mix well.
2. Season the ribs with salt and black pepper and then, coat with the liquid smoke. Now, rub the ribs with the Erythritol mixture.
3. Arrange the ribs onto the prepared baking sheet, meaty side down.
4. Arrange 2 layers of foil on top of ribs and then, roll and crimp edges tightly.
5. Bake for about 2-2½ hours or until desired doneness.
6. Remove the baking sheet from oven and place the ribs onto a cutting board.
7. Now, set the oven to broiler.
8. With a sharp knife, cut the ribs into serving-sized portions and evenly coat with the barbecue sauce.
9. Arrange the ribs onto a broiler pan, bony side up.
10. Broil for about 1-2 minutes per side. Remove from the oven and serve hot.

NUTRITION: Calories: 380 Cal Fat: 28 g Carbs: 8 g Protein: 14 g Fiber: 3 g

149. Valentine's Day Dinner

Preparation Time: 15'

Servings: 4

Cooking Time: 35'

Ingredients

- 1 tbsp. olive oil
- 4 large boneless rib pork chops
- 1 tsp. salt
- 1 cup of cremini mushrooms, chopped roughly
- 3 tbsps. yellow onion, chopped finely
- 2 tbsps. fresh rosemary, chopped
- 1/3 cups of homemade chicken broth
- 1 tbsp. Dijon mustard
- 1 tbsp. unsalted butter
- 2/3 cups of heavy cream
- 2 tbsps. sour cream

Directions

1. Heat the oil in a large skillet over medium heat and sear the chops with the salt for about 3-4 minutes or until browned completely.
2. With a slotted spoon, transfer the pork chops onto a plate and set aside.
3. In the same skillet, add the mushrooms, onion, and rosemary and sauté for about 3 minutes. Stir in the cooked chops, broth, and bring to a boil. Reduce the heat to low and cook, covered for about 20 minutes.
4. With a slotted spoon, transfer the pork chops onto a plate and set aside. In the skillet, stir in the butter until melted. Add the heavy cream and sour cream and stir until smooth. Stir in the cooked pork chops and cook for about 2-3 minutes or until heated completely.
5. Serve hot.

Nutrition: Calories: 400 Cal Fat: 21 g Carbs: 8 g Protein: 14 g Fiber: 5 g

150. Southeast Asian Steak Platter

Preparation Time: 15'		**Servings:** 4
	Cooking Time: 20'	

Ingredients

- 14 ozs. grass-fed sirloin steak, trimmed and cut into thin strips
- Freshly ground black pepper, to taste
- 2 tbsps. olive oil, divided
- 1 small yellow onion, chopped
- 2 garlic cloves, minced
- 1 Serrano pepper, seeded and chopped finely
- 3 cups of broccoli florets
- 3 tbsps. low-sodium soy sauce
- 2 tbsps. fresh lime juice

Directions

1. Season steak with black pepper.
2. In a large skillet, heat 1 tbsp. of the oil over medium heat and cook the steak for about 6-8 minutes or until browned from all sides.
3. Transfer the steak onto a plate.
4. In the same skillet, heat the remaining oil and sauté onion for about 3-4 minutes. Add the garlic and Serrano pepper and sauté for about 1 minute. Add broccoli and stir fry for about 2-3 minutes. Stir in cooked beef, soy sauce, and lime juice and cook for about 3-4 minutes.
5. Serve hot.

Nutrition: Calories: 418 Cal Fat: 30 g Carbs: 9 g Protein: 19 g Fiber: 5 g

151. Pesto flavored Steak

Preparation Time: 15'	Servings: 4

Cooking Time: 17'

Ingredients

- ¼ cup of fresh oregano, chopped
- 1½ tbsp. garlic, minced
- 1 tbsp. fresh lemon peel, grated
- ½ tsp. red pepper flakes, crushed
- Salt and freshly ground black pepper, to taste
- 1 lb. (1-inch thick) grass-fed boneless beef top sirloin steak
- 1 cup of. pesto
- ¼ cup of. feta cheese, crumbled

Directions

1. Preheat the gas grill to medium heat. Lightly, grease the grill grate.
2. In a bowl, add the oregano, garlic, lemon peel, red pepper flakes, salt, and black pepper and mix well.
3. Rub the garlic mixture onto the steak evenly.
4. Place the steak onto the grill and cook, covered for about 12-17 minutes, flipping occasionally.
5. Remove from the grill and place the steak onto a cutting board for about 5 minutes.
6. With a sharp knife, cut the steak into desired sized slices.
7. Divide the steak slices and pesto onto serving plates and serve with the topping of the feta cheese.
8. Serve hot.

Nutrition: Calories: 398 Cal Fat: 30 g Carbs: 9 g Protein: 19 g Fiber: 5 g

152. Flawless grilled Steak

Preparation Time:	21'		Servings:	5

	Cooking Time:	10'	

Ingredients

- ½ tsp. dried thyme, crushed
- ½ tsp. dried oregano, crushed
- 1 tsp. red chili powder
- ½ tsp. ground cumin
- ¼ tsp. garlic powder
- Salt and freshly ground black pepper, to taste
- 1½ lb. grass-fed flank steak, trimmed
- ¼ cup of Monterrey Jack cheese, crumbled

Directions

1. In a large bowl, add the dried herbs and spices and mix well.
2. Add the steaks and rub with mixture generously. Set aside for about 15-20 minutes. Preheat the grill to medium heat. Grease the grill grate. Place the steak onto the grill over medium coals and cook for about 17-21 minutes, flipping once halfway through. Remove the steak from the grill and place it onto a cutting board for about 10 minutes before slicing. With a sharp knife, cut the steak into desired sized slices.
3. Top with the cheese and serve.
4. Serve hot.

Nutrition: Calories: 271 Cal Fat: 32 g Carbs: 5 g Protein: 15 g Fiber: 5 g

153. Mongolian Beef

Preparation Time: 15′

Servings: 4

Cooking Time: 10′

Ingredients

- 1 lb. grass-fed flank steak, cut into thin slices against the grain
- 2 tsps. arrowroot starch
- Salt, to taste
- ¼ cup of avocado oil
- 1 (1-inch) piece fresh ginger, grated
- 4 garlic cloves, minced
- ½ tsp. red pepper flakes, crushed
- ¼ cup of water
- 1/3 cup of low-sodium soy sauce
- 1 tsp. red boat fish sauce
- 3 scallions, sliced
- 1 tsp. sesame seeds

Directions

1. In a bowl, add the steak slices, arrowroot starch, and salt and toss to coat well.
2. In a larger skillet, heat oil over medium-high heat and cook the steak slices for about 1½ minutes per side. With a slotted spoon, transfer the steak slices onto a plate. Drain the oil from the skillet but leaving about 1 tbsp. inside. In the same skillet, add the ginger, garlic, and red pepper flakes and sauté for about 1 minute.
3. Add the water, soy sauce, and fish sauce and stir to combine well.
4. Stir in the cooked steak slices and simmer for about 3 minutes.
5. Stir in the scallions and simmer for about 2 minutes.
6. Remove from the heat and serve hot with the garnishing of sesame seeds.
7. Serve hot.

Nutrition: Calories: 266 Cal Fat: 31 g Carbs: 6 g Protein: 16 g Fiber: 6 g

154. Sicilian Steak Pinwheel

Preparation Time: 15'

Servings: 6

Cooking Time: 35'

Ingredients

- 2 tbsps. dried oregano leaves
- 1/3 cup of fresh lemon juice
- 2 tbsps. olive oil
- 1 (2-lb.) grass-fed beef flank steak, pounded into ½-inch thickness.
- 1/3 cup of olive tapenade
- 1 cup frozen chopped spinach, thawed and squeezed
- ¼ cup feta cheese, crumbled
- 4 cups of fresh cherry tomatoes
- Salt, to taste

Directions

1. In a large baking dish, add the oregano, lemon juice, and oil and mix well.
2. Add the steak and coat with the marinade generously.
3. Refrigerate to marinate for about 4 hours, flipping occasionally.
4. Preheat the oven to 425 degrees F. Line a shallow baking dish with parchment paper.
5. Remove the steak from the baking dish, reserving the remaining marinade in a bowl.
6. Cover the bowl of marinade and refrigerate.
7. Arrange the steak onto a cutting board.
8. Place the tapenade onto the steak evenly and top with the spinach, followed by the feta cheese.
9. Carefully, roll the steak tightly to form a log.
10. With 6 kitchen string pieces, tie the log at 6 places.
11. Carefully, cut the log between strings into 6 equal pieces, leaving string in place.
12. In a bowl, add the reserved marinade, tomatoes, and salt and toss to coat.
13. Arrange the log pieces onto the prepared baking dish, cut-side up.
14. Now, arrange the tomatoes around the pinwheels evenly.
15. Bake for about 25-35 minutes.
16. Remove from the oven and set aside for about 5 minutes before serving.
17. Serve hot.

Nutrition: Calories: 3958 Cal Fat: 20 g Carbs: 7 g Protein: 19 g Fiber: 5 g

155. American Beef Wellington

PREPARATION TIME:	20'		SERVINGS:	4

COOKING TIME:	40'

INGREDIENTS

- 2 (4-ozs.) grass-fed beef tenderloin steaks, halved
- Salt and freshly ground black pepper, to taste
- 1 tbsp. butter
- 1 cup mozzarella cheese, shredded
- ½ cup of almond flour
- 4 tbsps. liver pate
-

DIRECTIONS

1. Preheat the oven to 400 degrees F. Grease a baking sheet.
2. Season the steaks with salt and black pepper evenly.
3. In a frying pan, melt the butter over medium-high heat and sear the beef steaks for about 2-3 minutes per side.
4. Remove from the heat and set aside to cool completely.
5. In a microwave-safe bowl, add the mozzarella cheese and microwave for about 1 minute.
6. Remove from the microwave and immediately, stir in the almond flour until a dough form.
7. Place the dough between 2 parchment paper pieces and with a rolling pin, roll to flatten it.
8. Remove the upper parchment paper piece.
9. Divide the rolled dough into 4 pieces.
10. Place 1 tbsp. of pate onto each dough piece and top with 1 steak piece.
11. Cover each steak piece with dough completely.
12. Arrange the covered steak pieces onto the prepared baking sheet in a single layer.
13. Bake for about 20-30 minutes or until the pastry is a golden brown.
14. Serve hot.

NUTRITION: Calories: 311 Cal Fat: 23 g Carbs: 5 g Protein: 25 g Fiber: 6 g

156. Pastry-free Beef Wellington

Preparation Time:	20'		Servings:	2

Cooking Time:	40'

Ingredients

For Duxelles:
- 2 tbsps. olive oil
- 3 large button mushrooms
- 1 tbsp. yellow onions, chopped
- 1 tsp. garlic powder
- Salt, to taste

For Filling:
- 8 thin prosciutto slices
- 1 (9-ozs.) grass-fed filet mignon
- Salt, to taste
- 2 tbsps. olive oil
- 1 tbsp. yellow mustard

Directions

1. Preheat the oven to 400 degrees F. Grease a baking sheet.
For duxelles:
2. In a food processor, add the mushrooms, onions, garlic, salt, and oil and pulse until pureed.
3. In a nonstick frying pan, add the pureed mixture over medium heat and cook for about 10 minutes, stirring frequently.
4. Remove from the heat and set aside.
5. Place a large piece of cling film onto a smooth surface.
6. Arrange the prosciutto slices over cling film, side-by-side form a rectangular layer, overlapping slightly.
7. Spread the duxelles over the prosciutto layer evenly.
8. Season the filet mignon with a little salt.
9. In a frying pan, heat the oil and sear the filet mignon for about 2 minutes per side.
10. Remove from the heat and place the filet mignon onto a plate.
11. Now, spread the mustard over the filet mignon evenly.
12. Arrange the filet mignon in the middle of the prosciutto and duxelles layer.
13. Carefully, wrap the prosciutto around the filet mignon.
14. Then wrap the cling-film around the package to secure it.
15. With the second piece of cling film, wrap the prosciutto-wrapped package tighter and refrigerate for about 15 minutes.
16. Remove the cling-film from the prosciutto-wrapped beef and arrange onto the prepared baking sheet.
17. Bake for 20-25 minutes.
18. Remove from the oven and cut the beef Wellington in 2 portions.
19. Serve hot.

Nutrition: Calories: 302 Cal Fat: 20 g Carbs: 9 g Protein: 23 g Fiber: 5 g

157 SUPER SALMON PARCEL

PREPARATION TIME: 15'

SERVINGS: 6

COOKING TIME: 20'

INGREDIENTS

- 6 (3-oz.) salmon fillets
- Salt and freshly ground black pepper, to taste
- 1 yellow bell pepper, seeded and cubed
- 1 red bell pepper, seeded and cubed
- 4 plum tomatoes, cubed
- 1 small yellow onion, sliced thinly
- ½ cup fresh parsley, chopped
- ¼ cup of olive oil
- 2 tbsps. fresh lemon juice

DIRECTIONS

1. Preheat the oven to 400 degrees F.
2. Arrange 6 pieces of foil onto a smooth surface. Place 1 salmon fillet onto each foil piece and sprinkle with salt and black pepper. In a bowl, add the bell peppers, tomato, and onion, and mix. Place veggie mixture over each fillet evenly and top with parsley. Drizzle with oil and lemon juice. Fold the foil around salmon mixture to seal it. Arrange the foil packets onto a large baking sheet in a single layer. Bake for about 20 minutes.
3. Serve hot.

NUTRITION: Calories: 418 Cal Fat: 30 g Carbs: 9 g Protein: 19 g Fiber: 5 g

158. New England Salmon Pie

PREPARATION TIME:	20'		SERVINGS:	5

COOKING TIME:	50'

INGREDIENTS

For Crust:
- ¾ C. almond flour
- 4 tbsps. coconut flour
- 4 tbsps. sesame seeds
- 1 tbsp. psyllium husk powder
- 1 tsp. organic baking powder
- Pinch of salt
- 1 organic egg
- 3 tbsps. olive oil
- 4 tbsps. water

For Filling:
- 8 ozs. smoked salmon
- 4¼ oz. cream cheese softened
- 1¼ cup cheddar cheese, shredded
- 1 cup of mayonnaise
- 3 organic eggs
- 2 tbsps. fresh dill, finely chopped
- ½ tsp. onion powder
- ¼ tsp. ground black pepper

DIRECTIONS

1. Preheat the oven to 350 degrees F. Line a 10-inch springform pan with parchment paper.
2. For the crust: place all the ingredients in a food processor, fitted with a plastic pastry blade, and pulse until a dough ball is formed.
3. Place the dough into prepared springform pan and with your fingers, gently press in the bottom.
4. Bake for about 12-15 minutes or until lightly browned.
5. Remove the pie crust from oven and let it cool slightly.
6. Meanwhile, for the filling: In a bowl add all the ingredients and mix well.
7. Place the cheese mixture over the pie crust evenly.
8. Bake for about 35 minutes or until the pie is golden brown.
9. Remove the pie from oven and let it cool slightly.
10. Cut into 5 equal-sized slices and serve warm.
11. Serve hot.

NUTRITION: Calories: 726 Cal Fat: 28 g Carbs: 8 g Protein: 18 g Fiber: 5 g

159. Keto Sausage Breakfast Sandwich

Preparation Time: 5'	**Servings:** 4
Cooking Time: 15'	

Ingredients

- 6 large eggs
- 2 tbsps. heavy cream
- Pinch red pepper flakes
- Kosher salt
- Freshly ground black pepper
- 1 tbsp. butter
- 3 slices cheddar
- 6 frozen sausage patties, heated according to package instructions
- Avocado, sliced

Directions

1. Beat the eggs, heavy cream, and red pepper flakes together in a small bowl.
2. Heat butter in a non-stick container over medium flame. Pour 1/3 of the eggs into your skillet. Place a cheese slice in the center and allow it to sit for about 1 minute. Fold the egg sides in the middle, covering the cheese. Remove from saucepan and repeat with eggs left over.
3. Serve the eggs with avocado in between two sausage patties.
4. Serve hot.

Nutrition: Calories: 128 Cal Fat: 31 g Carbs: 7 g Protein: 19 g Fiber: 5 g

160. Cabbage Hash Browns

Preparation Time: 10'

Servings: 2

Cooking Time: 25'

Ingredients

- 2 large eggs
- 1/2 tsp. garlic powder
- 1/2 tsp. kosher salt
- Freshly ground black pepper
- 2 cup shredded cabbage
- 1/4 small yellow onion, thinly sliced
- 1 tbsp. vegetable oil

Directions

1. Whisk shells, eggs, garlic powder, and salt together in a large bowl. Season with black potatoes. Add the chicken and onion to the mixture of the eggs and blend together.
2. Heat oil in a large skillet over medium to high heat. In the pan, divide the mixture into four patties and press to flatten with the spatula. Cook for about 3 minutes each side, until golden and tender.
3. Serve hot.

Nutrition: Calories: 167 Cal Fat: 23 g Carbs: 7 g Protein: 12 g Fiber: 4 g

161. Keto Breakfast Cups

Preparation Time: 15'

Servings: 12

Cooking Time: 40'

Ingredients

- 2 lbs. ground pork
- 1 tbsp. freshly chopped thyme
- 2 cloves garlic, minced
- 1/2 tsp. paprika
- 1/2 tsp. ground cumin
- 1 tsp. kosher salt
- Freshly ground black pepper
- 2 1/2 cups chopped fresh spinach
- 1 cup shredded white cheddar
- 12 eggs
- 1 tbsp. freshly chopped chives

Directions

1. Oven preheats to 400 ° c. combine the soiled pork, thyme, garlic, paprika, cumin, and salt in a large bowl. Season with peppers.
2. Attach a small handful of pork to each tin of muffin well then press the sides to make a cup. Spinach and cheese should be evenly divided between cups. Season with salt and pepper and crack an egg on top of each cup.
3. Bake for about 25 minutes, until eggs are set, and sausage is cooked through. Garnish and serve with chives.
4. Serve hot.

Nutrition: Calories: 418 Cal Fat: 30 g Carbs: 9 g Protein: 19 g Fiber: 5 g

162. Egg Salad Recipe

Preparation Time: 15'

Servings: 6

Cooking Time: 20'

Ingredients

- 3 tbsps. mayonnaise
- 3 tbsps. Greek yogurt
- 2 tbsps. red wine vinegar
- Kosher salt
- Freshly ground black pepper
- 8 hard-boiled eggs, cut into eight pieces, plus more for garnish
- 8 strips bacon, cooked and crumbled, plus more for garnish
- 1 avocado, thinly sliced
- 1/2 cup crumbled blue cheese, plus more for garnish
- 1/2 cup cherry tomatoes, halved, plus more for garnish
- 2 tbsps. freshly chopped chives

Directions

1. Stir mayonnaise, cream, and the red wine vinegar in a small bowl. Season with pepper and salt.
2. Kindly combine the eggs, bacon, avocado, blue cheese, and cherry tomatoes in a large serving bowl. Gradually fold in the mayonnaise dressing until the ingredients are coated slightly, then season with salt and pepper. Garnish with the chives and extra toppings.
3. Serve hot.

Nutrition: Calories: 204 Cal Fat: 31 g Carbs: 8 g Protein: 12 g Fiber: 3 g

163. Buffalo Shrimp Lettuce Wraps

PREPARATION TIME:	15′		SERVINGS:	4

COOKING TIME:	20′

INGREDIENTS

- 1/4 tbsp. butter
- 2 garlic cloves, minced
- 1/4 cup of hot sauce, such as Frank's
- 1 tbsp. extra-virgin olive oil
- 1 lb. shrimp, peeled and deveined, tails removed
- Kosher salt
- Freshly ground black pepper
- 1 head romaine leaf separated, for serving
- 1/4 red onion, finely chopped
- 1 rib celery, sliced thin
- 1/2 cup blue cheese, crumbled

DIRECTIONS

1. Make buffalo sauce: Melt butter over medium heat in a small saucepan. When completely melted, add the garlic and cook for 1 minute until it is fragrant. Attach hot sauce to combine, and stir. Switch heat to low while the shrimp are cooking.
2. Make shrimp: Heat oil in a large skillet over medium heat. Add shrimp, and add salt and pepper to season. Cook, flipping halfway, till both sides are pink and opaque, around 2 minutes per side turn off the heat and apply the sauce to the buffalo, tossing to coat.
3. Assemble wraps: add a small scoop of shrimp to a roman leaf center, then top with red onion, celery, and blue cheese.
4. Serve hot.

NUTRITION: Calories: 310 Cal Fat: 21 g Carbs: 7 g Protein: 17 g Fiber: 5 g

KETO DIET COOKBOOK *for women over 50*

164. Broccoli Bacon Salad

PREPARATION TIME: 15'		**SERVINGS:** 6
	COOKING TIME: 20'	

INGREDIENTS

Salad:
- Kosher salt
- 3 heads of broccoli, cut into bite-size pieces
- 2 carrots, shredded
- 1/2 red onion, thinly sliced
- 1/2 cup dried cranberries
- 1/2 cup sliced almonds
- 6 slices bacon, cooked and crumbled

Dressing:
- 1/2 cup of mayonnaise
- 3 tbsps. apple cider vinegar
- kosher salt
- Freshly ground black pepper

DIRECTIONS

1. Bring 4 cups of salted water up to a boil in a medium saucepan. Prepare a large bowl of ice water while waiting for the water to boil.
2. Add broccoli florets to the heated water, and cook for 1 to 2 minutes until tender. Remove with a slotted spoon and put the ice water in the prepared cup. Drain flourishes within a colander when cold.
3. Combine broccoli, red onion, carrots, cranberries, nuts, and bacon in a large bowl.
4. Whisk vinegar and mayonnaise together in a medium bowl and season with salt and pepper.
5. Pour the broccoli mixture over the dressing and stir to combine.
6. Serve hot.

NUTRITION: Calories: 301 Cal Fat: 27 g Carbs: 8 g Protein: 13 g Fiber: 5 g

165. Keto Bacon Sushi

| PREPARATION TIME: | 10' | | SERVINGS: | 12 |

| COOKING TIME: | 30' |

INGREDIENTS

- 6 slices bacon halved
- 2 Persian cucumbers, thinly sliced
- 2 medium carrots, thinly sliced
- 1 avocado, sliced
- 4 ozs. cream cheese softened
- Sesame seeds, for garnish

DIRECTIONS

1. Preheat oven to around 400o. Strip an aluminum foil baking sheet and fit it with a refrigerating rack. Lay the bacon halves in an even layer and bake for 11 to 13 minutes, until slightly crisp yet pliable.
2. In the meantime, the cucumbers, carrots, and avocado are sliced into parts around the bacon width.
3. Place one even layer of cream cheese on each slice when the bacon is cool enough to touch. Equally, divide vegetables between the bacon and put them on one end. Roll up tightly on vegetables.
4. Garnish, and serve with sesame seeds
5. Serve hot.

NUTRITION: Calories: 217 Cal Fat: 24 g Carbs: 7 g Protein: 12 g Fiber: 5 g

166. CAPRESE ZOODLES

PREPARATION TIME: 10'

SERVINGS: 4

COOKING TIME: 24'

INGREDIENTS

- 4 large zucchinis
- 2 tbsps. extra-virgin olive oil
- kosher salt
- Freshly ground black pepper
- 2 cups cherry tomatoes halved
- 1 cup mozzarella balls, quartered if large
- 1/4 cup fresh basil leaves
- 2 tbsps. balsamic vinegar

DIRECTIONS

1. Creating zoodles out of zucchini using a spiralizer.
2. In a large bowl, add the zoodles, mix with the olive oil, and season with the salt and pepper. Let them marinate for 15 minutes.
3. In zoodles, add the tomatoes, mozzarella, and basil and toss until combined.
4. Drizzle, and drink with balsamic.
5. Serve hot.

NUTRITION: Calories: 310 Cal Fat: 23 g Carbs: 8 g Protein: 13g Fiber: 5 g

167. Zucchini Sushi

PREPARATION TIME: 20'	SERVINGS: 4

COOKING TIME: 20'

Ingredients

- 2 medium zucchinis
- 4 ozs. cream cheese softened
- 1 tsp. Sriracha hot sauce
- 1 tsp. lime juice
- 1 cup lump crab meat
- 1/2 carrot, cut into thin matchsticks
- 1/2 avocado, diced
- 1/2 cucumber, cut into thin matchsticks
- 1 tsp. Toasted sesame seeds

Directions

1. Slice each zucchini into thin flat strips, using a vegetable peeler. Place the zucchini on a paper towel-lined plate to sit while the rest of your ingredients are prepared.
2. Combine cream cheese, sriracha, and lime juice in a medium-sized cup.
3. Place two slices of zucchini horizontally flat on a cutting board (so that the long side faces you). Place a lean layer of cream cheese over it, then top the left with a slice of lobster, carrot, avocado, and cucumber each.
4. Tightly roll up zucchini, starting from the left side. Repeat with slices and fillings of remaining zucchini. Before eating, sprinkle over sesame seeds.
5. Serve hot.

NUTRITION: Calories: 268 Cal Fat: 31 g Carbs: 4 g Protein: 13 g Fiber: 2 g

168. Basil Avocado Frail Salad Wraps & Sweet Potato Chips

PREPARATION TIME: 20'

SERVINGS: 4

COOKING TIME: 50'

INGREDIENTS

Sweet Potato Chips:
- Kosher salt
- Freshly ground black pepper
- Cooking spray
- 2 -3 medium potatoes, sliced into 1/8"-thick coins

Shrimp Salad
- 1/4 small red onion, finely diced
- 20 large frails, peeled and deveined (about 3/4 lb.)
- 1 1/2 cups halved grape tomatoes
- Cooking spray
- 2 avocados, diced
- 4 fresh basil leaves, thinly sliced
- 2 large heads butterhead or romaine lettuce

Marinade:
- Juice of 2 lemons
- 2 cloves garlic, minced
- 3 fresh basil leaves, thinly sliced
- 2 tbsps. white wine vinegar
- 3 tbsps. extra-virgin olive oil or avocado oil
- 1/2 tsp. paprika
- Kosher salt
- Freshly ground black pepper

NUTRITION: Calories: 419 Cal Fat: 28 g Carbs: 10 g Protein: 12 g Fiber: 5 g

DIRECTIONS

1. Make sweet potato chips: preheat the oven to 375o and grease the cooking spray on a large baking sheet. Arrange also a layer of sweet potatoes and season with salt and pepper.
2. Roast for 15 minutes, then flip and roast for 15 minutes, until crispy. Let them cool, then move to a re-sealable container until they are ready for eating.
3. In the meantime, make shrimp salad: grease a large skillet with cooking spray over medium heat. Add the shrimp and cook, occasionally stirring, for 2 minutes per side, until pink and no longer opaque. Set aside and let it cool down.
4. Create marinade: whisk the lemon juice, garlic, basil, vinegar, butter, and paprika together in a small bowl and season with salt and pepper.
5. Stir the tomatoes, onion, avocados, and basil together in a large bowl. Fold in the shrimps. Pour over shrimp salad and mix until covered.
6. Place the shrimp salad in a re-sealable container in the fridge. When ready to eat, serve them in lettuce cups.
7. Serve hot.

169. CALIFORNIA BURGER BOWLS

PREPARATION TIME: 10'

SERVINGS: 4

COOKING TIME: 20'

INGREDIENTS

- 1/2 up of extra-virgin olive oil
- 1/3 cup of balsamic vinegar
- 3 tbsps. Dijon mustard
- 2 tsps. honey
- 1 clove garlic, minced
- Kosher salt
- Freshly ground black pepper

Burger:
- 1 lb. grass-fed organic ground beef
- 1 tsp. Worcestershire sauce
- 1/2 tsp. chili powder
- 1/2 tsp. onion powder
- Kosher salt
- Freshly ground black pepper
- 1 package butterhead lettuce
- 1 medium red onion, cut into 1/4" rounds
- 1 avocado, sliced
- 2 Walmart Fresh medium slicing tomatoes, thinly sliced

DIRECTIONS

1. Make the dressing: whip together the dressing ingredients in a medium bowl.
2. Make burgers: mix beef and Worcestershire sauce, chili powder, and onion powder in another large bowl. Season with pepper and salt, then stir until just blended together. Form into four patties.
3. Heat a large grill pan over medium heat and then grill the onions until they are charred and tender, about 3 minutes each. Remove and detach burgers from the grill pan. Cook until sewn on both sides and cook for medium, around 4 minutes per side, to your taste.
4. Assemble: toss lettuce in a large bowl with 1/2 the dressing, and split between 4 bowls. Finish each with a patty burger, grilled onions, 1/4 slices of avocado, and tomatoes. Drizzle and help with remaining dressage and serve.
5. Serve hot.

NUTRITION: Calories: 312 Cal Fat: 29 g Carbs: 3 g Protein: 15 g Fiber: 6 g

170. Parmesan Brussels Sprouts Salad

Preparation Time:	25'		Servings:	6

	Cooking Time:	25'

Ingredients

- 5 tbsps. extra-virgin olive oil
- 5 tbsps. lemon juice
- 1/4 cup freshly chopped parsley
- Kosher salt
- Freshly ground black pepper
- 2 lbs. Brussels sprouts, halved and thinly sliced (about 8 cups)
- 1/2 cup chopped toasted almonds
- 1/2 cup pomegranate seeds
- Shaved Parmesan, for serving

Directions

1. Whisk olive oil, lemon juice, parsley, two teaspoons of salt, and one teaspoon of pepper in a medium bowl until combined.
2. Add the sprouts in Brussels and toss until fully coated.
3. Let sit, sometimes tossing, before serving for at least 20 minutes and up to 4 hours.
4. Until eating, fold in almonds and pomegranate seeds and garnish with a rasped parmesan.
5. Serve hot.

NUTRITION: Calories: 218 Cal Fat: 28 g Carbs: 4 g Protein: 14 g Fiber: 5 g

171. KETO QUESADILLAS

PREPARATION TIME: 10'

SERVINGS: 4

COOKING TIME: 35'

INGREDIENTS

- 1 tbsp. extra-virgin olive oil
- 1 bell pepper, sliced
- 1/2 yellow onion, sliced
- 1/2 tsp. chili powder
- Kosher salt
- Freshly ground black pepper
- 3 cups shredded Monterey Jack
- 3 cups shredded cheddar
- 4 cups shredded chicken
- 1 avocado, thinly sliced
- 1 green onion, thinly sliced
- Sour cream, for serving

DIRECTIONS

1. Preheat oven to 400o, and line two medium parchment paper baking sheets.
2. Heat oil on medium-high heat in a medium skillet. Add the onion and pepper and season with chili powder, salt, and pepper. Cook for 5 minutes, until tender. Move onto a platform.
3. Stir cheeses together in a medium-sized dish. Attach 1 1/2 cups of mixed cheese to the middle of both prepared baking sheets. Spread into an even surface, and form a circle, the size of a tortilla flour.
4. Bake the cheeses around the bottom, 8 to 10 minutes, until melty and slightly golden. Attach a mixture of onion-pepper, shredded chicken, and slices of avocado to one half each. Let them cool slightly, then use the parchment paper and a small spatula to raise and fold one side of the "tortilla" cheese gently over the side with the fillings. Return to heat on the oven, 3 to 4 more minutes. Repeat to add two quesadillas.
5. Split quarters of every quesadilla. Garnish before serving, with green onion and sour cream.

NUTRITION: Calories: 290 Cal Fat: 22 g Carbs: 4 g Protein: 14 g Fiber: 5 g

172. Keto stuffed Cabbage

Preparation Time: 15'

Servings: 12

Cooking Time: 45'

Ingredients

Sauce:
- 1 (14-oz.) can diced tomatoes
- 1 tbsp. apple cider vinegar
- 1/2 tsp. red pepper flakes
- 1 tsp. onion powder
- 1 tsp. garlic powder
- 1 tsp. dried oregano
- Kosher salt
- Freshly ground black pepper
- 1/4 cup of extra-virgin olive oil

Cabbage Rolls:
- 12 cabbage leaves
- 1 lb. ground beef
- 3/4 lb. ground pork
- 1 cup rice cauliflower
- 3 green onions, thinly sliced
- 1/4 cup chopped parsley, plus more for serving
- Freshly ground black pepper

Directions

Sauce:
1. Preheat the oven to 375° c. Puree tomatoes, in a blender, apple cider vinegar, red pepper flakes, onion powder, garlic powder and oregano; salt and pepper seasoning.
2. Heat oil in a large, deep pan (or big pot) over medium heat. Add the pureed tomato sauce, bring to a simmer then lower to medium-low, and cook for 20 minutes until thickened slightly.

Cabbage Rolls:
3. Flinch the cabbage leaves in a large pot of boiling water until tender and flexible, around 1 minute set aside
4. For the filling: mix 1⁄2 c in a large bowl. Tomato sauce, meat from the farm, cauliflower rice, scallions, and parsley. Top with pepper and salt.
5. Put a thin layer of sauce on a large baking dish underneath. Slice the hard-triangular rib out of each cabbage leaf using a paring knife. Place approximately 1⁄3 cup filling in one end of each leaf, then roll up and tuck into the sides as you move. Layer rolls in a baking dish to seam-side-down on top of the sauce. Remaining spoon sauce over the cabbage rolls. Bake until the meat is properly cooked through and the internal temperature hits 150 ° "4 for 45 minutes to 55 minutes. Apply more parsley to garnish before serving.

Nutrition: Calories: 229 Cal Fat: 20 g Carbs: 3 g Protein: 19 g Fiber: 3 g

173. Garlic Rosemary Pork Chops

PREPARATION TIME:	10'	**SERVINGS:**	4

COOKING TIME: 30'

INGREDIENTS

- 4 pork loin chops
- Kosher salt
- Freshly ground black pepper
- 1 tbsp. freshly minced rosemary
- 2 cloves garlic, minced
- 1/2 cup (1 stick) butter, melted
- 1 tbsp. extra-virgin olive oil

DIRECTIONS

1. Preheat the oven to 375° F. Spice the pork with salt and pepper generously.
2. Mix the butter, rosemary, and garlic together in a small bowl. Set aside.
3. Heat olive oil over medium-high flame, then places pork chops in an oven-safe skillet. Sear for 4 minutes until crispy, flip over and cook for 4 minutes. Clean the pork with garlic butter, generously.
4. Place the bucket in the oven and cook for 10-12 minutes until cooked (145° for medium). Serve with more butter over garlic.

NUTRITION: Calories: 390 Cal Fat: 30 g Carbs: 6 g Protein: 19g Fiber: 5 g

174. Lemon Butter Fish

Preparation Time: 10'

Servings: 6

Cooking Time: 20'

Ingredients

- 1 tbsp. lemon juice
- 4 tbsps. butter, unsalted
- Sea salt & pepper, to taste
- 2 tbsps. almond flour
- 2 tbsps. olive oil
- 2 tilapia fillets
- Sea salt & pepper, to taste

Directions

1. Warm the butter in a small pan over medium heat. Warm the butter until it's slightly browned.
2. Add the lemon juice, pepper, and salt and stir constantly. Adjust seasoning to taste. Set aside while you cook your fillets.
3. Rinse the fish fillets and pat them dry before sprinkling with salt and pepper.
4. Spread the flour on a plate or shallow dish and dredge the fillets, spreading the flour over the fillets as needed.
5. Heat a non-stick skillet over medium heat and warm the oil in it until it's shimmering.
6. Place the fillets in the pan and cook for about two minutes per side until golden and crisp on either side.
7. Remove the fish from the heat and place it on the plate. Drizzle the sauce over it and serve immediately!

Nutrition: Calories: 310 Cal Fat: 39 g Carbs: 5 g Protein: 14 g Fiber: 5 g

175. Chili Lime Cod

| PREPARATION TIME: | 10' | | SERVINGS: | 2 |

| COOKING TIME: | 10' |

INGREDIENTS

- 1/3 cup of coconut flour
- ½ tsp. cayenne pepper
- 1 egg, beaten
- 1 lime
- 1 tsp. crushed red pepper flakes
- 1 tsp. garlic powder
- 12 ozs. cod fillets
- Sea salt & pepper, to taste

DIRECTIONS

1. Preheat the oven to 400° Fahrenheit and line a baking sheet with non-stick foil.
2. Place the flour in a shallow dish (a plate works fine) and drag the fillets of cod through the beaten egg. Dredge the cod in the coconut flour, then lay on the baking sheet.
3. Sprinkle the tops of the fillets with the seasoning and lime juice.
4. Bake for 10 to 12 minutes until the fillets are flaky.
5. Serve immediately!

NUTRITION: Calories: 412 Cal Fat: 35 g Carbs: 6 g Protein: 13 g Fiber: 7 g

176. Lemon Garlic Shrimp Pasta

Preparation Time: 10'	**Servings:** 4

Cooking Time: 10'

Ingredients

- ½ lemon, thinly sliced
- ½ tsp. paprika
- 1 lb. "lg." lemon garlic shrimp, deveined & peeled
- 1 tsp. basil, fresh & chopped
- 14 oz. Miracle Noodle Angel Hair pasta
- 2 cloves garlic, minced
- 2 tbsps. butter
- 2 tbsps. extra virgin olive oil
- Sea salt & pepper, to taste

Directions

1. Drain the packages of Miracle noodles and rinse them under cool running water.
2. Bring a pot of water to a boil and place the noodles in the boiling water for two minutes before pulling them back out again.
3. Place the boiled noodles in a hot pan over medium heat and allow the excess moisture to cook off of them. Set aside.
4. Add the butter and olive oil to the pan, then add the garlic and stir.
5. Place the shrimp and the lemon slices in the pan and allow to cook until the shrimp is done, about three minutes per side.
6. Once the shrimp is done, add the salt, pepper, and paprika to the pan, then top with the noodles.
7. Toss to coat everything together, top with basil, and serve!

Nutrition: Calories: 360 Cal Fat: 21 g Carbs: 4 g Protein: 14 g Fiber: 5 g

177. One-Pan Tex Mex

Preparation Time: 5'

Servings: 4

Cooking Time: 10'

Ingredients

- 1/3 cup baby corn, canned
- 1/3 cup cilantro, chopped & separated
- ½ cup chicken stock
- ½ cup diced tomatoes & green chiles
- ½ tsp. garlic powder
- ½ tsp. oregano
- 1 tsp. cumin
- 2 cups cauliflower, riced
- 2 cups chicken breast, cooked & diced
- 2 cups Mexican cheese blend, shredded
- 2 tbsps. extra virgin olive oil
- 2 tsps. chili powder

Directions

1. Slice baby corn into small pieces and set aside. Press any liquid out of the riced cauliflower and set aside.
2. In a large pan over medium heat, warm your oil and sauté the cauliflower rice for about two minutes.
3. Add all ingredients except for the cheese and cilantro, and stir well to cook.
4. Stir in about half of the cilantro and allow the flavors to meld.
5. Stir about half the cheese into the mix and stir until melted and combined.
6. Serve and top with remaining cheese and cilantro for garnish!

Nutrition: Calories: 345 Cal Fat: 28 g Carbs: 7 g Protein: 17 g Fiber: 5 g

178. Spinach Artichoke-stuffed Chicken Breasts

Preparation Time: 15'

Servings: 6

Cooking Time: 15'

Ingredients

- ¼ cup Greek yogurt
- ¼ cup spinach, thawed & drained
- ½ cup artichoke hearts, thinly sliced
- ½ cup mozzarella cheese, shredded
- 1 ½ lb. chicken breasts
- 2 tbsps. olive oil
- 4 ozs. cream cheese
- Sea salt & pepper, to taste

Directions

1. Pound the chicken breasts to a thickness of about one inch. Using a sharp knife, slice a "pocket" into the side of each. This is where you will put the filling.
2. Sprinkle the breasts with salt and pepper and set aside.
3. In a medium bowl, combine cream cheese, yogurt, mozzarella, spinach, artichoke, salt, and pepper and mix thoroughly. A hand mixer may be the easiest way to combine all the ingredients thoroughly.
4. Spoon the mixture into the pockets of each breast and set aside while you heat a large skillet over medium heat and warm the oil in it. If you have an extra filling you can't fit into the breasts, set it aside until just before your chicken is done cooking.
5. Cook each breast for about eight minutes per side, then pull off the heat when it reaches an internal temperature of about 165° Fahrenheit.
6. Just before you pull the chicken out of the pan, heat the remaining filling to warm it through and to rid it of any cross-contamination from the chicken. Once hot, top the chicken breasts with it.
7. Serve!

Nutrition: Calories: 238 Cal Fat: 22 g Carbs: 5 g Protein: 17 g Fiber: 4 g

179. CHICKEN PARMESAN

| PREPARATION TIME: | 20' | | SERVINGS: | 4 |

| COOKING TIME: | 15' |

INGREDIENTS

- ¼ cup of avocado oil
- ¼ cup of almond flour
- ¼ cup parmesan cheese, grated
- ¾ cup of marinara sauce, sugar-free
- ¾ cup mozzarella cheese, shredded
- 2 eggs, beaten
- 2 tsps. Italian seasoning
- 3 oz. pork rinds, pulverized
- 4 lbs. chicken breasts, boneless & skinless
- Sea salt & pepper, to taste

DIRECTIONS

1. Preheat the oven to 450° Fahrenheit and grease a baking dish.
2. Place the beaten egg into one shallow dish. Place the almond flour in another. In a third dish, combine the pork rinds, parmesan, and Italian seasoning and mix well.
3. Pat the chicken breasts dry and pound them down to about ½" thick.
4. Dredge the chicken in the almond flour, then coat in egg, then coat in crumb.
5. Heat a large sauté pan over medium-high heat and warm oil until shimmering.
6. Once the oil is hot, lay the breasts into the pan and do not move them until they've had a chance to cook. Cook for about two minutes, then flip as gently as possible (a fish spatula is perfect) then cook for two more. Remove the pan from the heat.
7. Place the breasts in the greased baking dish and top with marinara sauce and mozzarella cheese.
8. Bake for about 10 minutes.
9. Serve!

NUTRITION: Calories: 621 Cal Fat: 24 g Carbs: 6 g Protein: 14 g Fiber: 6 g

180. Sheet Pan Jalapeño Burgers

Preparation Time: 10'

Servings: 4

Cooking Time: 20'

Ingredients

Burgers:
- 24 ozs. ground beef
- Sea salt & pepper, to taste
- ½ tsp. garlic powder
- 6 slices bacon, halved
- 1 med. onion, sliced into ¼ rounds
- 2 jalapeños, seeded & sliced
- 4 slices pepper jack cheese
- ¼ cup of mayonnaise
- 1 tbsp. chili sauce
- ½ tsp. Worcestershire sauce
- 8 lbs. leaves of Boston or butter lettuce
- 8 dill pickle chips

Directions

1. Preheat the oven to 425° Fahrenheit and line a baking sheet with non-stick foil.
2. Mix the salt, pepper, and garlic into the ground beef and form 4 patties out of it.
3. Line the burgers, bacon slices, jalapeño slices, and onion rounds onto the baking sheet and bake for about 18 minutes.
4. Top each patty with a piece of cheese and set the oven to boil.
5. Broil for 2 minutes, then remove the pan from the oven.
6. Serve one patty with 3 pieces of bacon, jalapeño slices, onion rounds, and desired amount of sauce with 2 pickle chips and 2 parts of lettuce.
7. Enjoy!

Nutrition: Calories: 608 Cal Fat: 29 g Carbs: 5 g Protein: 16 g Fiber: 4 g

181. GRILLED HERB GARLIC CHICKEN

PREPARATION TIME: 5'

SERVINGS: 2

COOKING TIME: 10'

INGREDIENTS

- 1 ¼ lb. chicken breasts, boneless & skinless - 1 tbsp. garlic & herb seasoning mix
- 2 tsps. extra virgin olive oil - Sea salt & pepper, to taste

DIRECTIONS

1. Heat a grill pan or your grill. Coat the chicken breasts in a little bit of olive oil and then sprinkle the seasoning mixture onto them, rubbing it in. Cook the chicken for about eight minutes per side and make sure the chicken has reached an internal temperature of 165°. Serve hot with your favorite sides!

NUTRITION: Calories: 187 Cal Fat: 24 gCarbs: 5 g Protein: 12 g Fiber: 4 g

182. Blackened Salmon with Avocado Salsa

Preparation Time: 30'

Servings: 6

Cooking Time: 21'

Ingredients

- 1 tbsp. extra virgin olive oil
- 4 filets of salmon (about 6 ozs. each)
- 4 tsps. Cajun seasoning
- 2 med. avocados, diced
- 1 cup cucumber, diced
- ¼ cup red onion, diced
- 1 tbsp. parsley, chopped
- 1 tbsp. lime juice
- Sea salt & pepper, to taste

Directions

1. Heat a skillet over medium-high heat and warm the oil in it.
2. Rub the Cajun seasoning into the fillets, then lay them into the bottom of the skillet once it's hot enough.
3. Cook until a dark crust forms, then flip and repeat.
4. In a medium mixing bowl, combine all the ingredients for the salsa and set aside.
5. Plate the fillets and top with ¼ of the salsa yielded.
6. Enjoy!

Nutrition: Calories: 445 Cal Fat: 31 g Carbs: 6 g Protein: 10 g Fiber: 5 g

183. Delectable Tomato Slices

Preparation Time:	15'		Servings:	10

Cooking Time:	15'

Ingredients

- ½ cup of. mayonnaise
- ½ cup of. ricotta cheese, shredded
- ½ cup part-skim mozzarella cheese, shredded
- ½ cup of parmesan and Romano cheese blend, grated
- 1 tsp. garlic, minced
- 1 tbsp. dried oregano, crushed
- Salt, to taste
- 4 large tomatoes, cut each one in 5 slices

Directions

1. Preheat the oven to broiler on high. Arrange a rack about 3-inch from the heating element.
2. In a bowl, add the mayonnaise, cheeses, garlic, oregano, and salt and mix until well combined and smooth.
3. Spread the cheese mixture over each tomato slice evenly.
4. Arrange the tomato slices onto a broiler pan in a single layer.
5. Broil for about 3-5 minutes or until the top becomes golden brown.
6. Remove from the oven and transfer the tomato slices onto a platter.
7. Set aside to cool slightly.
8. Serve warm.

NUTRITION: Calories: 110 Cal Fat: 29 g Carbs: 2 g Protein: 16 g Fiber: 5 g

184. Grain-free Tortilla Chips

PREPARATION TIME: 15'

SERVINGS: 6

COOKING TIME: 16'

INGREDIENTS

- 1½ cup mozzarella cheese, shredded
- ½ cup of almond flour
- 1 tbsp. golden flaxseed meal
- Salt and freshly ground black pepper, to taste

DIRECTIONS

1. Preheat the oven to 375o F. Line 2 large baking sheets with parchment paper.
2. In a microwave-safe bowl, add the cheese and microwave for about 1 minute, stirring after every 15 seconds.
3. In the bowl of melted cheese, add the almond flour, flaxseed meal, salt, and black pepper and with a fork, mix well.
4. With your hands, knead until a dough form.
5. Make 2 equal sized balls from the dough.
6. Place 1 dough ball onto each prepared baking sheet and roll into an 8x10-inch rectangle.
7. Cut each dough rectangle into triangle-shaped chips.
8. Arrange the chips in a single layer.
9. Bake for about 10-15 minutes, flipping once halfway through.
10. Remove from oven and set aside to cool before serving.

NUTRITION: Calories: 80 Cal Fat: 14 g Carbs: 6 g Protein: 13 g Fiber: 4 g

185. Cheeses Chips

Preparation Time: 15'

Servings: 8

Cooking Time: 15'

Ingredients

- 3 tbsps. coconut flour
- ½ cup strong cheddar cheese, grated and divided
- ¼ cup Parmesan cheese, grated
- 2 tbsps. butter, melted
- 1 organic egg
- 1 tsp. fresh thyme leaves, minced

Directions

1. Preheat the oven to 350o F. Line a large baking sheet with parchment paper.
2. In a bowl, place the coconut flour, ¼ cup of grated cheddar, Parmesan, butter, and egg and mix until well combined.
3. Set the mixture aside for about 3-5 minutes.
4. Make 8 equal-sized balls from the mixture.
5. Arrange the balls onto the prepared baking sheet in a single layer about 2-inch apart.
6. With your hands, press each ball into a little flat disc.
7. Sprinkle each disc with the remaining cheddar, followed by thyme.
8. Bake for about 13-15 minutes or until the edges become golden brown.
9. Remove from the oven and let them cool completely before serving.

Nutrition: Calories: 189 Cal Fat: 28 g Carbs: 4 g Protein: 14 g Fiber: 5 g

186. Snack Parties Treat

PREPARATION TIME: 10'	**SERVINGS:** 4

COOKING TIME: 6'

INGREDIENTS

- 8 bacon slices
- 8 mozzarella cheese sticks, frozen overnight
- 1 cup of. olive oil

DIRECTIONS

1. Wrap a bacon slice around each cheese stick and secure it with a toothpick.
2. In a cast-iron skillet, heat the oil over medium heat and fry the mozzarella sticks in 2 batches for about 2-3 minutes or until golden brown from all sides.
3. With a slotted spoon, transfer the mozzarella sticks onto a paper towel-lined plate to drain.
4. Set aside to cool slightly.
5. Serve warm.

NUTRITION: Calories: 119 Cal Fat: 22g Carbs: 3 g Protein: 11 g Fiber: 5 g

187. SWEET TOOTH CARVING PANA COTTA

| PREPARATION TIME: | 15' | | SERVINGS: | 4 |

| COOKING TIME: | 5' |

INGREDIENTS

- 1½ cup of. unsweetened almond milk, divided
- 1 tbsp. unflavored powdered gelatin
- 1 cup of. unsweetened coconut milk
- 1/3 cup of swerve
- 3 tbsps. cacao powder
- 2 tsps. instant coffee granules
- 6 drops liquid stevia

DIRECTIONS

1. In a large bowl, add ½ C. of almond milk and sprinkle evenly with gelatin.
2. Set aside until soaked.
3. In a pan, add the remaining almond milk, coconut milk, Swerve, cacao powder, coffee granules, and stevia and bring to a gentle boil, stirring continuously.
4. Remove from the heat.
5. In a blender, add the gelatin mixture, and hot milk mixture and pulse until smooth.
6. Transfer the mixture into serving glasses and set aside to cool completely.
7. With plastic wrap, cover each glass and refrigerate for about 3-4 hours before serving.

NUTRITION: Calories: 293 Cal Fat: 17 g Carbs: 5 g Protein: 16 g Fiber: 7 g

188. Halloween special Fat Bombs

Preparation Time: 15'

Servings: 24

Cooking Time: 3'

Ingredients

- 4 ozs. cream cheese softened
- ½ cup of coconut oil
- ½ cup of homemade pumpkin puree
- ¼ cup of. monk fruit sweetener
- 2 tsps. pumpkin pie spice
- ½ cup of. pecans, toasted
- ¼ tsp. ground cinnamon

Directions

1. In a medium pan, add the cream cheese and coconut oil over medium-low heat and cook for about 2-3 minutes or until smooth, stirring continuously.
2. Remove from the heat and transfer the cream cheese mixture into a bowl.
3. Add the pumpkin puree, monk fruit sweetener, and pumpkin pie spice and with an electric mixer, beat until well combined.
4. Place the mixture into 24 silicone molds evenly.
5. Top each mold with the pecans, and sprinkle with cinnamon.
6. Freeze the molds for about 4 hours before serving.

Nutrition: Calories: 76 Cal Fat: 10 g Carbs: 2 g Protein: 2 g Fiber: 3 g

189. Breakfast Toast in a Bowl

Preparation Time: 15'	**Servings:** 4

Cooking Time: 30'

Ingredients

- 4 tbsps. butter + greasing
- 1 tbsp. chopped fresh basil
- 12 salami slices
- 8 tomato slices
- 4 low-carb bread slices
- 4 eggs
- Salt and black pepper to taste

Directions

1. Preheat the oven to 300°F/150°C.
2. Heat 1 tablespoon of butter in a skillet over medium heat and sauté the basil until fragrant. Stir in the salami and cook for 3 minutes per side or until golden brown. Remove the salami and basil to a plate and set aside.
3. Put the tomatoes in the pan and cook for 3 to 5 minutes per side or until brown around the edges.
4. Brush 4 medium ramekins with some butter and press a bread slice into each bowl to line the walls of the ramekins. If the bread tears in the middle, that's okay.
5. Place one salami each in the center of each bread and then two salamis each against the walls of the ramekin that doesn't have complete bread covering. The goal is to create a cup of food in the ramekins either with bread or salami.
6. Divide the tomatoes into the bread cup and crack an egg into the center of the food cup. Bake in the oven until the egg whites set but the yolks still running.
7. Take out the ramekins, season with salt, black pepper, and serve immediately.

Nutrition: Calories: 310 Cal Fat: 28 g Carbs: 4 g Protein: 14 g Fiber: 5 g

190. Cocoa and Berry Breakfast Bowl

PREPARATION TIME: 10'		**SERVINGS:** 2
	COOKING TIME: 0'	

INGREDIENTS

- ½ cup (113.5 g) strawberries, fresh or frozen
- ½ cup (113.5 g) blueberries, fresh or frozen
- 1 cup (240 ml) unsweetened almond milk
- Sugar-free maple syrup to taste
- 2 tbsps. unsweetened cocoa powder
- 1 tbsp. cashew nuts for topping

DIRECTIONS

1. Divide the berries into 4 serving bowls and pour on the almond milk.
2. Drizzle with the maple syrup and sprinkle the cocoa powder on top, a tablespoon per bowl.
3. Top with the cashew nuts and enjoy immediately.

NUTRITION: Calories: 298 Cal Fat: 23 g Carbs: 4 g Protein: 12 g Fiber: 3 g

191. Turmeric Nut Loaf with Zesty Cream Cheese

Preparation Time: 25'

Servings: 6

Cooking Time: 45'

Ingredients

- 4 eggs, separated
- 1 cup (160 g) swerve sugar, divided
- 1 stick (100 g) butter, room temperature
- ½ tsp salt, divided
- ½ cup (113.5g) almond flour
- ½ cup (113.5g) ground almonds
- 1 tsp turmeric powder + extra for garnish
- A pinch cinnamon powder
- 1 tsp baking powders
- 1 tsp fresh lemon zest
- 1 tbsp. plain vinegar
- 3 tbsps. sugar-free maple syrup
- 7 ozs. (200 g) cream cheese

Directions

1. Preheat the oven to 350°F/175°C and line a loaf pan with grease-proof paper. Set aside.
2. Using electric beaters, whisk the egg whites and half of the swerve sugar until stiff.
3. Add the remaining swerve sugar, butter, salt, and whisk until smooth.
4. Pour in the egg yolks, almond flour, ground almonds, turmeric powder, cinnamon powder, baking powder, lemon zest, and two-thirds of the vinegar. Mix until smooth batter forms.
5. Pour the batter into the loaf pan and level the top with a spatula. Bake for 45 minutes or until a small skewer inserted comes out with moist crumbs and no wet batter.
6. Remove the pan and allow the bread to cool in the pan.
7. Meanwhile, in a medium bowl, mix the maple syrup, cream cheese, and remaining vinegar until smooth.
8. Remove the bread onto a cutting board and spread the topping on top. Garnish with the lemon zest and pistachios. Slice and serve.

Nutrition: Calories: 573 Cal Fat: 26 g Carbs: 4 g Protein: 18 g Fiber: 5 g

192. Herby Goat Cheese Frittata

Preparation Time: 15'

Servings: 6

Cooking Time: 16'

Ingredients

- 1 tbsp. avocado oil for frying
- 2 ozs. (56 g) bacon slices, chopped
- 1 medium red bell pepper, deseeded and chopped
- 1 small yellow onion, chopped
- 2 scallions, chopped
- 1 tbsp. chopped fresh chives
- Salt and black pepper to taste
- 8 eggs, beaten
- 1 tbsp. unsweetened almond milk
- 1 tbsp. chopped fresh parsley
- 3 ½ ozs. (100 g) goat cheese, divided
- ¾ oz. (20 g) grated Parmesan cheese

Directions

1. Preheat the oven to 350°F/175°C.
2. Heat the avocado oil in a medium cast-iron pan and cook the bacon for 5 minutes or until golden brown. Stir in the bell pepper, onion, scallions, and chives. Cook for 3 to 4 minutes or until the vegetables soften. Season with salt and black pepper.
3. In a bowl, beat the eggs with the almond milk and parsley. Pour the mixture over the vegetables, stirring to spread out well. Share half of the goat cheese on top.
4. Once the eggs start to set, divide the remaining goat cheese on top, season with salt, black pepper, and place the pan in the oven. Bake for 5 to 6 minutes or until the eggs set all around.
5. Take out the pan, scatter the Parmesan cheese on top, slice, and serve warm.

Nutrition: Calories: 494 Cal Fat: 27g Carbs: 5 g Protein: 19 g Fiber: 5 g

193. Chocolate American Pancakes

Preparation Time:	15'	**Servings:**	4

Cooking Time: 12'

Ingredients

- 2 cups (250 g) almond flour
- 2 tsps. baking powder
- 2 tbsps. erythritol
- ¾ tsp salt
- 2 eggs
- 1 1/3 cups (320 ml) almond milk
- 2 tbsps. butter + more for frying

Topping:
- 2 tbsps. unsweetened chocolate buttons
- Sugar-free maple syrup
- 4 tbsps. semi-salted butter

Directions

1. In a medium bowl, mix the almond flour, baking powder, erythritol, and salt.
2. Whisk the eggs, almond milk, and butter in another bowl. Add the mixture to the dry ingredients and combine until smooth.
3. Melt about 1 ½ tablespoon of butter in a non-stick skillet, pour in portions of the batter to make small circles, about 2 pieces per batch (approximately ¼ cup of batter each.) Sprinkle some chocolate buttons on top and cook for 1 to 2 minutes or until set beneath. Turn the pancakes and cook for 1 more minute or until set.
4. Remove the pancakes onto a plate and make more with the remaining ingredients. Work with more butter and reduce the heat as needed to prevent sticking and burning.
5. Drizzle the pancakes with some maple syrup, top with more butter (as desired,) and enjoy!

Nutrition: Calories: 294 Cal Fat: 29 g Carbs: 5 g Protein: 18 g Fiber: 7 g

194. Green Shakshuka

Preparation Time: 25'

Servings: 6

Cooking Time: 25'

Ingredients

- 1 tbsp. olive oil
- 2 tbsps. almond oil
- ½ medium green bell pepper, deseeded and chopped
- 1 celery stalk, chopped
- ¼ cup (57 g) green beans, chopped
- 1 garlic clove, minced
- 2 tbsps. fresh mint leaves
- 3 tbsps. fresh parsley leaves
- ½ cup (113 g) baby kale
- ¼ tsp plain vinegar
- Salt and black pepper to taste
- ¼ tsp nutmeg powder
- 7 ozs. (200 g) feta cheese, divided
- 4 eggs

Directions

1. Heat the olive oil and almond oil in a medium frying pan over medium heat.
2. Add the bell pepper, celery, green beans, and sauté for 5 minutes or until the vegetables soften.
3. Stir in the garlic, mint leaves, 2 tablespoons of parsley, and cook until fragrant, 1 minute.
4. Add the kale, vinegar, and mix. Once the kale starts wilting, season with salt, black pepper, nutmeg powder, and stir in half of the feta cheese. Cook for 1 to 2 minutes.
5. After, use the spatula to create four holes in the food and crack an egg into each hole. Cook until the egg whites set but the yolks still running. Season the eggs with salt and black pepper.
6. Turn the heat off and scatter the remaining feta cheese on top. Garnish with the remaining parsley and serve the shakshuka immediately.

Nutrition: Calories: 322 Cal Fat: 21 g Carbs: 6 g Protein: 11 g Fiber: 2 g

195. Eggs and Cheddar Breakfast Burritos

Preparation Time: 15'

Servings: 4

Cooking Time: 6'

Ingredients

- 3 tbsps. butter
- 2 small yellow onions, chopped
- ½ medium orange bell pepper, deseeded and chopped
- 10 eggs, beaten
- Salt and black pepper to taste
- 8 tbsps. grated cheddar cheese (white and sharp)
- 4 (8-inch) low-carb soft tortillas
- 2 tbsps. chopped fresh scallions
- Hot sauce for serving

Directions

1. Melt the butter in a skillet over medium heat and stir-fry the onions and bell pepper for 3 minutes or until softened.
2. Pour the eggs into the pan, let set for 15 seconds and then, scramble. Season with salt, black pepper, and stir in the cheddar cheese. Cook until the cheese melts.
3. Layout the tortillas, divide the eggs on top, and sprinkle some scallions and hot sauce on top. Fold two edges of each tortilla in and tightly roll the other ends over the filling. Slice into halves and enjoy the burritos.

Nutrition: Calories: 478 Cal Fat: 27 g Carbs: 7 g Protein: 14 g Fiber: 5 g

196. Cheesy Guacamole with Veggie Sticks

Preparation Time: 10'

Servings: 4

Cooking Time: 0'

Ingredients

- 12 avocados, peeled and pitted
- ½ small tomato, diced
- 1 tbsp. chopped fresh cilantro
- 1 green chili, deseeded and minced
- 1 tsp cumin powder
- 1 ½ cups grated cheddar cheese
- 3 tbsps. butter
- 1 tsp. vinegar
- Salt and black pepper to taste
- 2 celery stick, cut into thirds
- 1 small sweet red bell pepper, deseeded and julienned

Directions

1. Mash the avocado in a bowl using a fork or masher until smooth.
2. Mix in the tomatoes, cilantro, green chili, cumin powder, cheddar cheese, butter, vinegar, salt, and black pepper.
3. Serve the guacamole with the celery sticks and bell pepper strips. Enjoy!

Nutrition: Carbs: 6 g Protein: 17 g Fiber: 8 g Calories: 307 Cal Fat: 28 g

197. Cheese Patties with Raspberry Dip

Preparation Time: 15'

Servings: 4

Cooking Time: 4'

Ingredients

Cheesecakes:
- 1 2/3 cup (400 g) goat cheese
- 1/3 cup (68 g) grated Monterey Jack cheese
- 2 egg yolks
- ¼ cup (50 g) swerve sugar
- ½ cup (100 g) almond flour
- 2 tbsps. (30 g) xanthan gum
- 1 tsp (10 g) vanilla extract
- 3 tbsps. olive oil for frying

Raspberry Dip:
- 1 cup (200 g) fresh raspberries
- 2 tbsps. swerve sugar
- Mint leaves for garnish

Directions

Cheesecakes:
1. In a bowl, mix the goat cheese, Monterey Jack cheese, egg yolks, swerve sugar, almond flour, xanthan gum, and vanilla until well-combined. Shape the mixture into a dough and divide it into 6 to 8 (2-inch thick) patties.
2. Heat the olive oil in a non-stick skillet over low heat, and fry the cheese patties on both sides for 1 to 2 minutes per side or until golden brown and compacted.
3. Remove the cheesecakes to a paper towel-lined plate to drain grease and set aside.

Raspberry Dip:
4. 1 In a food processor, add the raspberries, swerve sugar, and blend until smooth.
5. Pour the mixture into a serving bowl, garnish with the mint leaves and enjoy with the cheesecakes.

Nutrition: Calories: 284 Cal Fat: 21 g Carbs: 5 g Protein: 17 g Fiber: 3 g

198. Tempura Zucchinis with Cream Cheese Dip

Preparation Time: 5'

Servings: 64

Cooking Time: 10'

Ingredients

Tempura Zucchinis:
- 1 ½ cups (200 g) almond flour
- 2 tbsps. heavy cream
- 1 tsp salt
- 2 tbsps. olive oil + extra for frying
- 1 ¼ cups (300 ml) water
- ½ tbsp. sugar-free maple syrup
- 2 large zucchinis, cut into 1-inch thick strips

Cream Cheese Dip:
- 8 ozs. cream cheese, room temperature
- ½ cup (113 g) sour cream
- 1 tsp taco seasoning
- 1 scallion, chopped
- 1 green chili, deseeded and minced

Directions

Tempura Zucchinis:
1. In a bowl, mix the almond flour, heavy cream, salt, peanut oil, water, and maple syrup.
2. Dredge the zucchini strips in the mixture until well-coated.
3. Heat about 4 tablespoons of olive oil in a non-stick skillet. Working in batches, use tongs to remove the zucchinis (draining extra liquid) into the oil. Fry per side for 1 to 2 minutes and remove the zucchinis onto a paper towel-lined plate to drain grease.
4. Enjoy the zucchinis.

Cream Cheese Dip:
5. In a bowl, mix the cream cheese, sour cream, taco seasoning, scallion, and green chili.
6. Serve the tempura zucchinis with the cream cheese dip.

Nutrition: Calories: 303 Cal Fat: 27 g Carbs: 6 g Protein: 17g Fiber: 2 gg

199. CHEESE FONDUE WITH LOW-CARB CROUTONS

PREPARATION TIME: 15'

SERVINGS: 4

COOKING TIME: 15'

INGREDIENTS

- 1 garlic clove, halved
- 1 cup (227 g) dry white wine
- 14 ozs (400 g) grated Mexican cheese blend
- 10 ozs. (283 g) grated Monterey Jack cheese
- 10 ozs. (283 g) grated cheddar cheese (white and sharp)
- 1 tbsp. fresh vinegar
- ¼ tsp nutmeg powder
- Black pepper to taste
- 1 tbsp. xanthan gum mixed with 2 drops of water
- 3 tbsps. butter
- 1 low-carb bread loaf, cut into 1-inch cubes

DIRECTIONS

1. Rub the inner part of a pot with the garlic and pour in the white wine. Cook over low heat until warm.
2. Slowly add the cheeses while gently stirring in one direction until the cheeses melt.
3. Stir in the vinegar, nutmeg powder, and black pepper.
4. If the mixture is too thin, add the xanthan gum and stir in the same direction until thickened. Pour the cheese fondue into a serving bowl and set aside for serving.
5. Melt the butter in a skillet and toast the bread cubes on both sides until golden brown and slightly crunchy.
6. Serve the cheese fondue with the low-carb bread pieces.

NUTRITION: Calories: 114 Cal Fat: 95 g Carbs: 12 g Protein: 69g Fiber: 0 g

200. Cold Avocado & Green Beans Soup

PREPARATION TIME:	15'		SERVINGS:	12

COOKING TIME:	11'

INGREDIENTS

- 1 tbsp. butter
- 2 tbsps. almond oil
- 1 garlic clove, minced
- 1 cup (227 g) green beans (fresh or frozen)
- ¼ avocado
- 1 cup heavy cream
- ½ cup grated cheddar cheese + extra for garnish
- ½ tsp. coconut aminos
- Salt to taste

DIRECTIONS

1. Heat the butter and almond oil in a large skillet and sauté the garlic for 30 seconds. Add the green beans and stir-fry for 10 minutes or until tender.
2. Add the mixture to a food processor and top with the avocado, heavy cream, cheddar cheese, coconut aminos, and salt. Blend the ingredients until smooth.
3. 3 Pour the soup into serving bowls, cover with plastic wraps and chill in the fridge for at least 2 hours.
4. Enjoy afterward with a garnish of grated white sharp cheddar cheese

NUTRITION: Calories: 230 Cal Fat: 20 g Carbs: 5 g Protein: 20 g Fiber: 2 g

Conclusion

Routines ware very important on this diet, and it's something that will help you stay healthy. As such, in this part, we are going to be giving you tips and tricks to make this diet work better for you and help you get an idea of routines that you can put in place for yourself.

Tip number one that is so important is "drink water!" This is absolutely vital for any diet that you're on, and you need it if not on one as well. However, this vital tip is crucial on a keto diet because when you are eating fewer carbs, you are storing less water, meaning that you are going to get dehydrated very easily. You should aim for more than the daily amount of water; however, remember that drinking too much water can be fatal as your kidneys can only handle so much as once. While this has mostly happened to soldiers in the military, it does happen to dieters as well, so it is something to be aware of.

Along with that same tip is to keep your electrolytes. You have three major electrolytes in your body. When you are on a keto diet, your body is reducing the amount of water that you store. It can be flushing out the electrolytes that your body needs as well, and this can make you sick. Some of the ways that you can battle this is by either salting your food or drinking bone broth. You can also eat pickled vegetables. Eat when you're hungry instead of snacking or eating constantly. This is also going to help, and when you focus on natural foods and health foods, this will help you even more. Eating foods that are processed is the worst thing you can do for fighting cravings, so you should really get into the routine of trying to eat whole foods instead. Another routine that you can get into is setting a note somewhere that you can see it that will remind you of why you're doing this in the first place and why it's important to you. Dieting is hard, and you will have moments of weakness where you're wondering why you are doing this. Having a reminder will help you feel better, and it can really help with your perspective.

KETO DIET COOKBOOK *for women over 50*

Tracking progress is something that straddles the fence. A lot of people say that this helps a lot of people and you can celebrate your wins, however, as everyone is different and they have different goals, progress can be slower in some than others. This can cause others to be frustrated and sad, as well as wanting to give up. One of the very most important things to remember is that while progress takes time, and you shouldn't get discouraged if you don't see results right away. With most diets, it takes at least a month to see any results. So, don't get discouraged and keep trying if your body is saying that you can. If you can't, then you will need to talk to your doctor and see if something else is for you.

You should make it a daily or everyday routine to try and lower your stress. Stress will not allow you to get into ketosis, which is that state that keto wants to put you in. The reason for this being that stress increases the hormone known as cortisol in your blood, and it will prevent your body from being able to burn fats for energy. This is because your body has too much sugar in your blood. If you're going through a really high period of stress right now in your life, then this diet is not a great idea. Some great ideas for this would be getting into the habit or routine of taking the time to do something relaxing, like walking and making sure that you're getting enough sleep, leads to the following routine that you need to do.

You need to get enough sleep. This is so important not just for your diet but also for your mind and body as well. Poor sleep also raises those stress hormones that can cause issues for you, so you need to get into the routine of getting seven hours of sleep at night on the minimum and nine hours if you can. If you're getting less than this, you need to change the routine you have in place right now and make sure that you establish a new routine where you are getting more sleep. As a result, your health and diet will be better.